The *Special K*
Challenge™
& Beyond

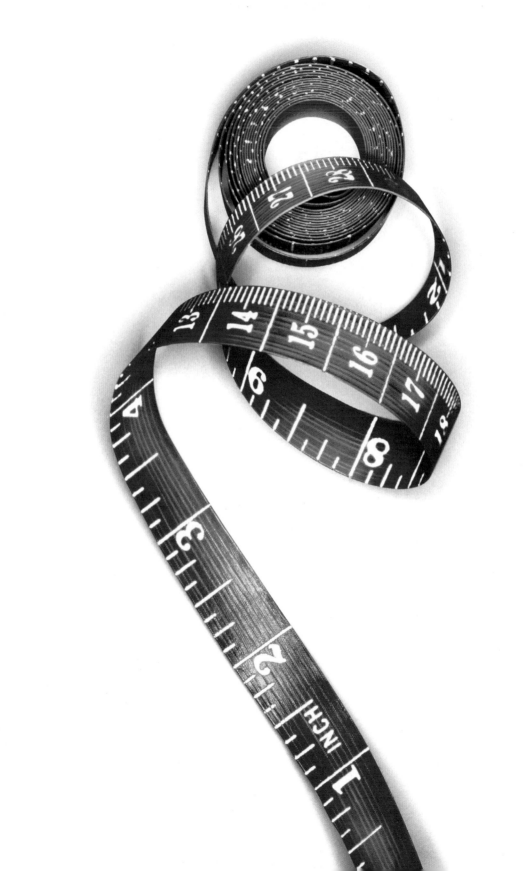

Kellogg's®

The *Special K*
Challenge™
& Beyond

Your guide to
weight management, healthy
living & delicious cooking

Foreword by Katherine Brooking, MS, RD

weldon**owen**

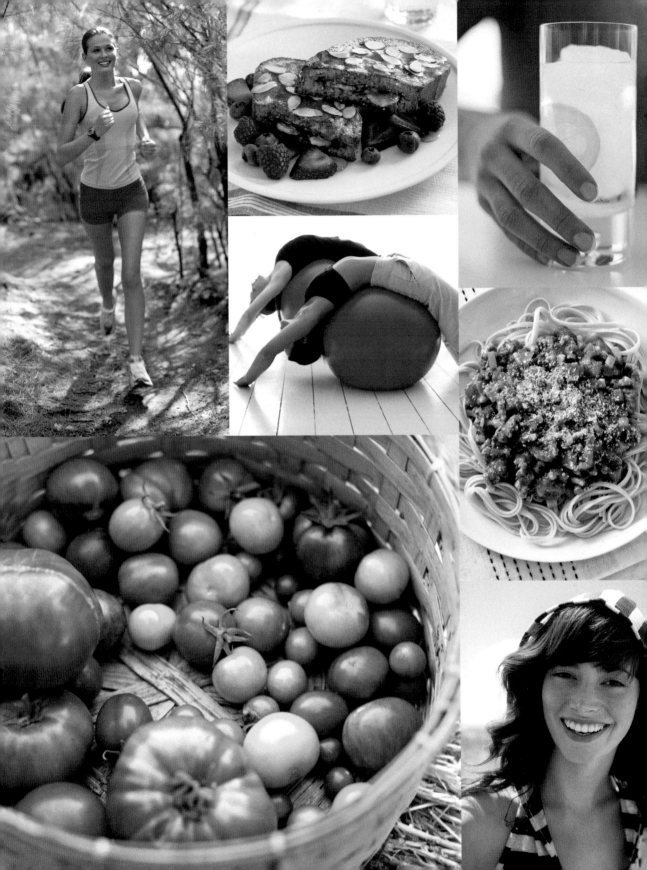

contents

Foreword

As a registered dietitian, I believe that the words "wholesome" and "delicious" can go hand in hand, and I often write and speak about how a healthy lifestyle starts right in your own kitchen. But let's face it: if food doesn't taste good, no matter how chock full of vitamins and minerals it may be, you won't want to eat it. That's why I was thrilled to hear that Kellogg Company was planning a cookbook and guide to living well that is packed with tasty, satisfying meals and loads of inspiration to help women both achieve their weight-management goals as well as maintain an enduringly healthy way of life.

Whether you are trying to lose weight, or simply want to cook balanced, portion-controlled meals that are in line with your wellness goals, this book provides everything you need. It begins with a brief primer on **The Special K Challenge,™** showing how to customize the two-week program to your own daily routine, but then goes well beyond. A special section covers the myriad ways to support your overall wellness including setting—and sticking to—your personal weight-management goals; nutrition basics; how to snack sensibly; tips for finding a fitness routine that works for you; relaxation and stress-reduction techniques; strategies for dealing with temptations; keeping a food journal; the basics of healthful cooking; and much more.

Next are 100 delicious and easy recipes for every meal of the day that will satisfy both your taste buds and your waistline. Many of the recipes offer bonus features on the health benefits of certain foods; suggestions for accompaniments to make recipes into full, healthful meals; and tips on customizing the recipes to your personal taste with wholesome ingredient substitutions.

I have always believed that a healthy way of life is within everyone's reach and I strive in my own work to help people make smart choices without feeling deprived. With this book as your guide, I believe that you, too, will discover that healthy living—and all the benefits that it provides—can be a reality.

Here's to your health and well-being!

Katherine Brooking, MS, RD

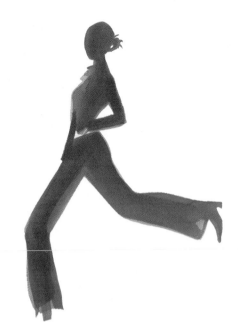

Help Manage Your Weight with Special K® Foods

A personal commitment to managing your weight is one of the most important—and positive—decisions you can make in your life. Start out on that journey and you can see results right away. You will notice the numbers on the scale drop; watch those inches fall on your tape measure; fit into your swimsuit; or drop a jeans or dress size.

These are all victories you deserve to achieve and celebrate. They're victories that become more possible with the help of **Special K** foods. We're here to be your weight-management partner, and that's the reason behind this book. On the following pages, you'll find practical, supportive information and advice to help you achieve your personal weight-management goal for results that can last a lifetime. You'll also discover how simple it can be to get a kick-start towards your goal with the help of the two-week-long **Special K Challenge™**. (Consult your physician before starting any diet or exercise program. Average weight loss when replacing meals with two cereal meals is 4.8 pounds. Average waist circumference reduction when replacing meals with two cereal meals is 1.3 inches. Weight loss may vary.)

We'll also share easy ways to cook and eat healthfully every day of the year with more than 100 delicious, satisfying, kitchen-tested recipes. You'll find helpful advice for adding enjoyable exercise to your daily life, which will burn calories and trim and tone your body. We'll also show you how, by nourishing your mind and spirit, you can manage your weight more successfully and more fully enjoy all the benefits that come from doing so. Just think what you could achieve with the help of this book:

YOU COULD ENJOY GREATER HEALTH Medical studies have shown that there's a direct relationship between maintaining a healthy weight and reducing your risk of diseases such as diabetes, cardiovascular disease, cancer and other illnesses.

YOU COULD LIVE A LONGER, MORE ACTIVE LIFE People who manage their weight find they have more energy, so they're able to do much more in their everyday life. The delicious foods you'll be eating will help you achieve and maintain a healthy weight and will boost your energy level.

YOU COULD FEEL MORE CONFIDENT AND CONTENT Any great victory in your life has the power to lift your spirits, making you feel confident and happy. Just imagine how great you could feel when you achieve and maintain your own weight-management goals, showing the world your very best self.

Simple changes for big success

Think of your own weight management journey as a series of single, simple daily steps toward a goal, and you can achieve victory easily and enjoyably. Here are just some of the things you'll discover how to do in this book:

Get a kick-start (page 13) Take **The Special K Challenge™** and after 2 weeks you could see real, positive changes in how you look and feel.

Eat more healthfully every day (page 24) Add delicious, easy-to-find treats to daily meals and feel more satisfied and more energetic.

Snack smart (page 32) Yes! Eating yummy, nutritious snacks on a regular basis can help you control hunger—and lose weight.

Enjoy exercise (page 38) Who said exercise should only happen at the gym? Move in whatever way makes you happy.

Incorporate relaxation (page 47) Moments of peace and quiet can help make weight management so much easier.

Cook delicious food (pages 54–63) Review the basics of healthy cooking, then start cooking and enjoying the recipes on pages 65–231.

Setting and Achieving Your Goals

When you begin your lifetime weight-management journey, you'll enjoy greater success by setting some simple goals and taking some easy steps that can help you maintain a healthy lifestyle. The few tips below, along with other ideas and insights we share throughout this book, will help you achieve victory.

MAKE FEELING GOOD YOUR MAIN MOTIVATION Instead of waiting for numbers to drop on your scale, look for real benefits you can see and feel in your everyday life. Do you have more energy? Do your clothes fit more comfortably? Do you feel more relaxed and in control? Savor such moments and you'll enjoy a true sense of victory regardless of what the scale might say. (See the opposite page for other methods you can use to measure your progress.)

BANISH THE WORD "DIET" The very thought of "dieting" carries all sorts of bad connotations. Long-term fad diets that focus exclusively on certain ingredients or eliminate any of the essential food groups (page 24) can leave you feeling unsatisfied—or worse. Such diets can deprive your body of essential nutrients because they lack variety. A better way to maintain a healthy weight successfully is to develop sensible, well-balanced eating habits that can last a lifetime.

LOSE WEIGHT SLOWLY AND STEADILY You didn't reach your current weight overnight. So, after you've given yourself a proven, responsible kick-start with **The Special K Challenge™,** it makes sense to take the time to lose weight gradually. Pounds that disappear rapidly may be water weight or result from starving yourself or exercising so rigorously that you simply cannot maintain the routine. In the case of weight management, the old saying is true: Slow and steady *does* win the race.

SET REALISTIC GOALS A high weight-loss goal can make you feel overwhelmed. Set shorter-term goals that feel achievable, like a certain reasonable percentage (for example, five percent) of your total body weight, and you'll set yourself up for success. (For more on setting fitness goals, turn to page 40.)

EXPECT VICTORY As you take small steps and make simple changes, remember: A positive attitude can help you achieve victory. Know that you can do it, small step by small step, simple change by simple change. Even if you have occasional slip-ups, you can and will reach your goal.

TRACK YOUR PROGRESS

According to the National Weight Control Registry (www.NWCR.ws), three-quarters of people who are successful at long-term weight management weigh themselves at least once a week. There are several other good ways to measure your progress:

Weigh in weekly

Weight can vary naturally from day to day. Over several days or a week, however, such fluctuations tend to level out. Your actual weight loss (or gain) is more likely to add up and register on the scale from one week to the next. It gives you a real sense of triumph if you've lost, or an indication that you need to be more diligent. For the most accurate indication of change, weigh yourself at the same time of day.

Measure your waist circumference

Without sucking in your stomach, measure your waist at your navel and write down the number. According to numerous studies, including one published in the August 2010 Archives of Internal Medicine, the smaller your waist, the lower your risk for early heart disease, high blood pressure and type 2 diabetes. Health risks increase if your waist is greater than 35 inches for women, or 40 inches for men. Keep track of your waist circumference, measuring it every time you've lost five or ten pounds.

Determine your BMI

Health care professionals use Body Mass Index (BMI) to calculate total body fat based on height and weight. To figure out your BMI, first multiply your weight in pounds by 703. Next, divide that figure by your height in inches. Finally, divide once again by your height. A BMI between 18.5 and 24.9 is considered healthy. A BMI over 25 is considered overweight, except for cases in which the extra weight is muscle. Keep track of your own BMI, recalculating it every time you've lost five or ten pounds.

Consult a professional

Your doctor, registered dietitian, personal trainer certified in weight management or a online resource from your health care provider can help you set a realistic target for your weight-management goals.

The Special K Challenge™

For years now, **The Special K Challenge** has helped women everywhere who want to lose an inch from their waists (and up to six pounds) in just two weeks*. On the following pages, you'll find detailed instructions for this easy-to-follow plan, including reasons for taking **The Special K Challenge** (pages 14–15), ideas for customizing it to your life (pages 18–19), suggestions for the third meal (page 17) and a quick-reference guide to the basics (page 16). In two weeks, victory can be yours!

*Consult your physician before starting any diet or exercise program. Average weight loss when replacing meals with two cereal meals is 4.8 pounds. Average waist circumference reduction when replacing meals with two cereal meals is 1.3 inches. Weight loss may vary.

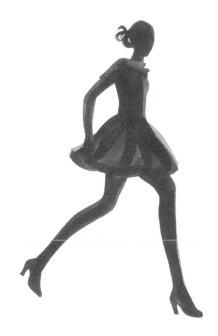

Reasons to Take The Special K Challenge™

There are three main times of year when most women take **The Special K Challenge.** These tend to be the seasons when they especially want to look their best or manage their weight more carefully, including resolution time right after the new year, the spring approach of summer's swimsuit season, and the fall leading up to the holiday season. With the help of **The Special K Challenge,** it becomes possible and even fun to trim down a bit, shape up and get ready for whatever life brings your way.

SLIM DOWN FOR RESOLUTION TIME Come January, many people resolve to manage their weight and eat more healthfully. In fact, countless surveys show that goals like getting fit, losing weight and living a healthier life consistently rank among the top three New Year's resolutions. **The Special K Challenge** provides an effective, reliable and easy way to get your resolution off to a great start.

GET LEAN FOR SWIMSUIT SEASON When the weather starts to warm up halfway through springtime, many women start thinking about fitting into last year's swimsuits or the new ones they'd like to buy. Trimming and toning yourself to get ready for swimsuit season can be a powerful motivator to start managing your weight. **The Special K Challenge** can give you the gentle support you need to get back into the swim of things.

DROP A JEANS SIZE FOR FALL Many women find that fall is the time of year they want to drop a jeans size, and **The Special K Challenge™** is a proven way to accomplish that goal.* You might find that dropping a jeans size is one of the easiest ways to feel good about yourself before the cool weather arrives.

Beyond these three times, of course, there are many other life occasions for which **The Special K Challenge** offers a proven way to give yourself a gentle, effective push toward your weight-management goals. Three popular reasons are:

REUNIONS Want to lose a few pounds before the big high school, college or family reunion? Many women make the grade with **The Special K Challenge.**

WEDDINGS Whether you're the bride-to-be, a member of the wedding party or simply a guest invited to the celebration, **The Special K Challenge** can take the anxiety out of getting ready for the big day.

PRE-HOLIDAYS One of the easiest ways to get ready for all the tempting foods and drinks offered during the festive season is to lose an inch, or up to six pounds,* before all the parties start. That way, not only will you be able to enjoy a bite of the seasonal treats every now and then, but you'll also look great in your favorite holiday outfit.

What's your own reason to get started on a lifetime of successful weight management? Whatever your answer, you'll discover a plan here that can help.

Using The Special K Challenge™ *wisely*

When you have successfully completed **The Special K Challenge** and achieved your own very specific short-term goal, you'll feel better about yourself. You'll feel victorious. But don't try to turn it into a full-time eating regimen. Instead, think of **The Special K Challenge** as an occasional kick-start, part of your long-range weight-management strategy that includes a wide variety of nutritious meals.

Consult your physician before starting any diet or exercise program. Average weight loss when replacing meals with two cereal meals is 4.8 pounds. Average waist circumference reduction when replacing meals with two cereal meals is 1.3 inches. Weight loss may vary.

SPECIAL K CHALLENGE™ BASICS

MEAL 1

Start your day sensibly

Eat any **Special K**® cereal with ¾ cup skim milk and your choice of fruit. (If eating **Special K** Low-Fat Granola, enjoy it with your choice of either milk or fruit.) Or, try a **Special K** Protein Shake or Protein Meal Bar.

MEAL 2

Refuel wisely

Replace a second meal with one of the following:

- A serving of **Special K** cereal, as outlined in Meal 1
- **Special K** Protein Meal Bar
- **Special K** Protein Shake

MEAL 3

Savor a healthful meal

Enjoy a wholesome meal using one of the recipes in this book, or your own creation, keeping it at or below 700 calories. Remember, you can make this "third meal" either the first, second, or last meal of the day, depending on your preference and lifestyle.

SNACK 4

Snack shrewdly

Enjoy two great-tasting snacks throughout the day

- **Special K** Protein Snack Bars
- **Special K** Cereal Bars
- **Special K** Crackers
- **Special K** Fruit Crisps
- **Special K** Cracker Chips
- **Special K** Protein Water Mixes

ENJOY FRUITS AND VEGGIES AS EXTRA SNACKS. ENJOY NON-CALORIC DRINKS AS USUAL.

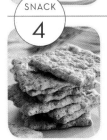

Enjoying Your Third Meal

Many women who take **The Special K Challenge**™ for the first time—and even some who are returning to kick-start their weight-management goals—are surprised by how much they are free to eat for their third meal, whether they make that meal their breakfast, lunch or dinner. But when you look at the numbers, it all makes perfect sense: A serving of **Special K**® cereal with skim milk, fruit, and coffee or tea—or a serving of a **Special K** protein meal bar or protein shake—gives you a satisfying, nutritious meal. Enjoy two such meals on **The Special K Challenge,** add two **Special K** snacks (plus fruit and vegetable snacks as desired) and you can still enjoy a satisfying, sensible and healthful third meal—and lose weight!* This book has plenty of advice on healthful eating (pages 24–35) and healthy cooking (pages 54–63) to help you get the best results while on **The Special K Challenge.**

PLANNING THE MENU We've designed many of the recipes in this book as third meal options while on **The Special K Challenge.** As you'll see, each of those recipes has a calorie count far lower than the 700 or so you can allow for your third meal, which means that you have plenty of flexibility to round out the meal with sensible portions of healthful appetizers, soups, salads, vegetables, grains, or even desserts; you'll find great recipes here for those, too. You'll also discover that these recipes yield multiple portions of delicious, tempting food that anyone can enjoy. With the help of this book, you can cook delicious, healthful food for your family and friends—and even entertain—or store and enjoy leftovers for another meal.

The third meal and beyond

The recipes in this book have been created to work not just for the third meal, but also well beyond the two-week **Special K Challenge.** There are a wide range of healthful meal options—and even some snacks—with dishes for all kinds of occasions throughout the year. Once you've completed **The Special K Challenge,** you can continue to find support and inspiration from this book to help you achieve your long-term weight-management goals. The recipes will work equally well for you whether you want to continue shedding pounds and trimming inches or to maintain a healthy weight.

Consult your physician before starting any diet or exercise program. Average weight loss when replacing meals with two cereal meals is 4.8 pounds. Average waist circumference reduction when replacing meals with two cereal meals is 1.3 inches. Weight loss may vary.

YOUR CUSTOM SPECIAL K CHALLENGE™

The **Special K Challenge** is easy—just follow the simple instructions outlined on page 16. Before you start, pick a version of the plan that best fits your own lifestyle, such as one of the four examples below. Remember, too, that with the help of a wide range of **Special K®** foods, there are many ways to customize the eating plan to your tastes and lifestyle. (Visit SpecialK.com for more creative ideas to make **The Special K Challenge** your own.)

Classic plan

You like the basics, the tried-and-true crowd pleasers. Here's a plan that's simple, easy and good for:

- People who want the essentials
- People who love the classics

The Strategy For two meals a day, enjoy classic **Special K** cereals and popular **Special K** foods like French Vanilla Protein Shakes and Chocolate Peanut Butter Protein Meal Bars.

The Third Meal Enjoy classic healthful recipes like Cheese Ravioli with Chunky Marinara Sauce (page 181), Easy Chicken Potpies (page 138), or Beef Stew with Mushrooms (page 163).

Snacks Between meals, enjoy favorite **Special K** snacks like Multi-Grain Crackers or Strawberry Cereal Bars.

On-the-go-plan

You're always running from A to B and back again. This portable, easy plan works well for:

- Busy moms
- Business travelers

The Strategy For two meals a day, enjoy your favorite **Special K** cereals whenever possible. At other times, rely on convenient, easy to carry **Special K** protein meal bars and protein shakes.

The Third Meal Look for the many delicious recipes in this book that are quick and easy to prepare, such as Seared Steak Salad (page 161), Ginger and Soy Salmon (page 102), or Oven-Fried Chicken Cutlets (page 133).

Snacks For nibbling, bring along whichever **Special K** snack bars or cereal bars appeal to you.

Chocolate-lovers' plan

Celebrate one of the most wonderful foods in the world. This plan is made for:

- Chocoholics
- Eaters with serious sweet tooths

The Strategy For your two meals a day, stock up on **Special K®** Chocolatey Delight cereal and Milk Chocolate Protein Shakes, plus any other varieties that appeal to you.

The Third Meal You may enjoy healthful dishes with a touch of fruity sweetness, such as Banana-Stuffed Multigrain French Toast (page 74), Orange-Glazed Stuffed Turkey Breast (page 150), or Pork Stew with Root Vegetables and Dried Fruits (page 175).

Snacks Munch on an array of chocolate flavors in **Special K** cereal bars and protein snack bars between meals.

Mix-it-up plan

You love to try new things. Designed to keep you interested, this plan is perfect for:

- People who get bored easily
- People who love variety

The Strategy Stock up on as many **Special K** cereals, shakes, and protein meal bars that sound appealing to you, and enjoy a different one for each of your two meals a day throughout the two weeks of **The Special K Challenge™**.

The Third Meal Keep your taste buds engaged with a variety of ethnic-influenced dishes, from Sichuan Orange Beef-and-Broccoli Stir-Fry (page 158) to Jamaican Chicken Breast with Mashed Sweet Potatoes (page 140) to Sautéed Shrimp Tacos (page 116).

Snacks Vary your snacks so you don't get bored. Between meals, enjoy a wide variety of **Special K** snack bars.

*Consult your physician before starting any diet or exercise program. Average weight loss when replacing meals with two cereal meals is 4.8 pounds. Average waist circumference reduction when replacing meals with two cereal meals is 1.3 inches. Weight loss may vary.

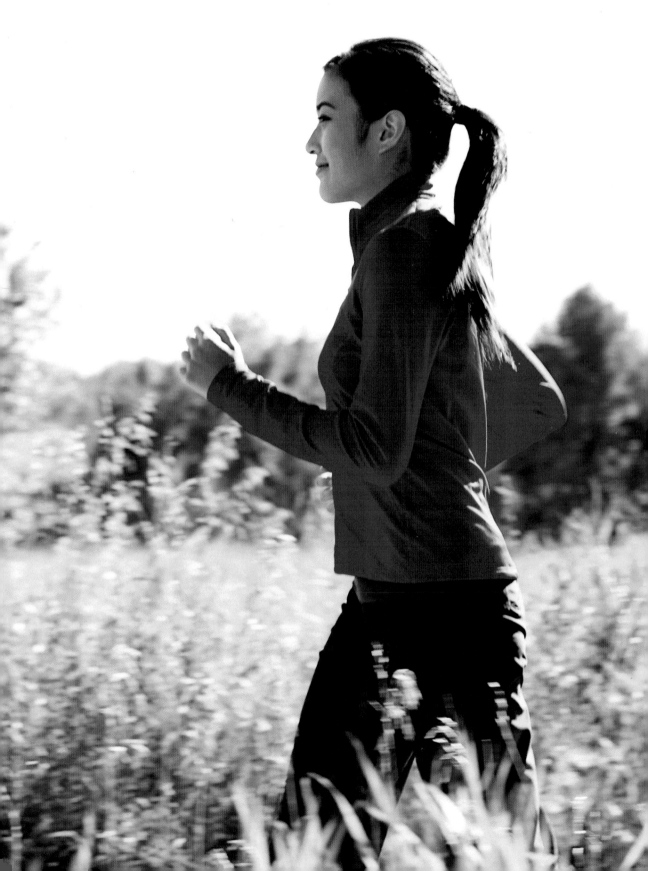

Beyond The Special K Challenge™

Congratulations! You've successfully completed

The Special K Challenge and you may have experienced

results that you can not only feel, but also that you, and the people

around you, can see. But how do you continue to achieve and maintain

your weight-management goals in the future? Consider the pages

that follow to be your road map to victory. In them you will find nutrition

basics, healthy eating guidelines, exercise tips and more. You'll

also discover all kinds of sensible and inspiring ways to support your

weight-management goals by nourishing your mind and spirit.

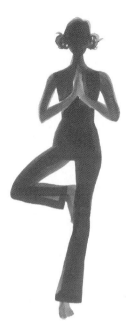

Three Steps to Reaching Your Goal

Your journey to long-term weight management consists of three phases: eating healthfully, exercising regularly, and nourishing your mind and spirit.

LEARN TO EAT SENSIBLY Your journey begins on pages 24–35, where you'll find an explanation of the basics of nutrition and healthful eating. You'll learn what it really means to enjoy a wholesome, well-balanced eating plan—and how easily you can tailor a plan to your own needs with the help of the U.S. Department of Agriculture's MyPyramid. You'll also find out how, by choosing nutritious, delicious foods that leave you feeling comfortably satisfied, you can more easily avoid overeating. Changing the way you think and behave around food is an important part of successful weight management. Here, you'll find plenty of tips for slowing down and savoring what you eat; keeping meals exciting through variety; and staying on track successfully when eating in restaurants, while traveling or during special celebrations. Let's be frank: Managing your weight is easier when the food you eat is tasty and satisfying. That's why the information on pages 54–63 focuses on the basics of planning and cooking healthful meals that you'll really enjoy eating. On pages 65–231 you will be able to put your newfound knowledge to the test with 100 tempting recipes. Each one has been kitchen-tested and includes a nutritional analysis to help you reach your personal weight-management goals.

EXERCISE FOR WEIGHT MANAGEMENT To manage your weight successfully, be sure to exercise regularly. The information on pages 36–41 will show you how easy and how much fun it can be to do just that. You'll learn about the different categories of exercise—stretching, cardiovascular workouts and strength training—and how each of these can not only help you achieve your weight-management goal, but also contribute to your general sense of well-being. You'll discover ways to "mix it up," keeping your regular exercise fresh and fun while also maximizing the benefits you get. And, most importantly, you'll find out simple strategies you can use to help you stick with an exercise plan, wherever you are and whatever you're doing.

FIND SUPPORT THROUGH MIND AND SPIRIT You may have noticed that even when topics deal with hard scientific fact—like nutrition basics or cardiovascular exercise—the mention of how you "feel" about healthy eating or regular exercise is never far away. That's because successful weight management also depends on supporting yourself through mind and spirit. The information on pages 42–53 will help you enlist both in achieving your goal. You'll learn easy ways to stay on track through support groups, meditation or simple relaxation and daily journaling.

Many ways to achieve victory

The pages that follow are packed with smart tips for lifelong weight management. Here are some examples:

Practice mindful eating (pages 30–31) Develop the habit of savoring your food bite by bite and you may discover you're eating less.

Snack, snack, snack! (pages 32–33) Sensible nibbling between meals can keep you energetic and satisfied while avoiding overeating.

Mix up your exercise (pages 38–39) Get more benefits from your physical activity by spicing it up with variety.

Picture yourself beautiful (page 43) Imagining yourself fit and healthy may help you achieve weight-management success.

"Fry" in your oven (page 60) Enjoy crunchy "fried" food without all the fat of deep-frying.

Keep turning the pages for more inspiration!

MYPYRAMID

The U.S. Department of Agriculture's (USDA's) MyPyramid is a handy tool for anyone who wants advice—specific or general—on healthful eating, offering simple guidelines on what and how much to eat from each of the basic food groups to help you maintain a healthy weight and keep your body working at its peak. It also helps you tailor your meals to your lifestyle and suggests how much exercise you need every day. Below is a summary of the USDA's powerful tool, including daily recommended serving amounts for women 19 to 50 years old. For more detailed information and any updates on how to use MyPyramid to achieve your weight management goals, visit www.MyPyramid.gov.

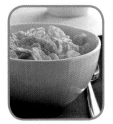

Grains 6 OUNCES, AT LEAST HALF AS WHOLE GRAINS

Whenever possible, choose whole-grain foods with fiber over refined grains. If you aren't yet eating many whole grains, try substituting brown rice for half of your usual white rice. Or replace 1 slice of white bread with 1 slice of whole-grain bread when you make a sandwich. **Ounce equivalents include:** 1 cup dry cereal (such as **Special K®** cereal); ½ cup cooked cereal; 1 slice bread; or ½ cup cooked pasta.

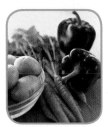

Vegetables 2½ CUPS

You can pack your plate with veggies. They're low in calories, rich in nutrients, and they fill you up, leaving you comfortably satisfied. Always add some frozen vegetables to canned soups or to frozen dinners; these convenience foods rarely include enough veggies. **One cup of vegetables is equal to:** 1 cup raw or cooked vegetables; 1 cup vegetable juice; or 2 cups raw leafy greens.

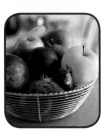

Fruits 2 CUPS (19-30 YEARS); 1½ CUPS (31-50 YEARS)

Keep whole fruits washed and within easy reach on your kitchen counter. Keep more fragile fruit in your fridge to use as toppings for cereal or yogurt. **One cup of fruit is equal to:** 1 cup bite-sized whole fruit; 1 cup cut-up fruit; 1 small piece of whole fruit such as a tangerine, a kiwi or a small apple; 1 cup 100% fruit juice; or ½ cup dried fruit.

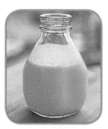

Milk & dairy 3 CUPS A DAY

Dairy foods are great sources of nutrients. Plenty of foods contain calcium, but nondairy sources generally contain less—and don't provide as much protein. An afternoon cup of hot cocoa made with nonfat milk and sugar-free cocoa mix is nutrient-rich and satisfying. **One cup of milk is equal to:** 1 cup milk or yogurt; or 1½ ounces natural cheese or 2 ounces processed cheese.

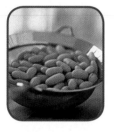

Meat & beans 5½ OUNCES (19-30 YEARS); 5 OUNCES (31-50 YEARS)

Choose low-fat or lean options more often. Go meatless one meal a week. Beans are a bonus because they're packed with satiating fiber and will count as a serving from both the vegetable group and the meat and beans group. **Ounce equivalents include:** 1 ounce meat, poultry, or fish; ¼ cup cooked beans; 1 egg; 1 tablespoon peanut butter; ½ ounce nuts or seeds.

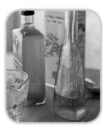

Oils 6 TEASPOONS (19-30 YEARS); 5 TEASPOONS (31-50 YEARS)

Oils and fats play an important role in a healthy diet. The best choices are those highest in monounsaturated fats like olive oil and canola oil, and polyunsaturated fats, like corn, soybean and safflower oils. Limit saturated fats, usually in solid form at room temperature, like butter or lard; and those containing unhealthy trans-fats such as margarine.

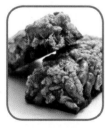

Discretionary calories 195 TO 360 CALORIES

This number is your remaining daily calorie budget, which is based on your age and how physically active you are. It can be used for "splurges" like sweets, sauces, beverages, or higher-fat foods. But remember: 195 to 360 calories isn't a lot. If you overdo it today, be sure to cut back or get more physical activity tomorrow.

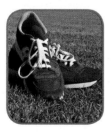

Physical activity AT LEAST 30 MINUTES A DAY

If you want a larger discretionary calories budget, do whatever gets your heart pumping (pages 36–41). If you have children, remember that they should get 60 minutes of exercise daily, so find fun ways to get the family moving together—from sports to a walk in the park to an old-fashioned game of tag.

Benefits of a Healthful Diet

By following the simple daily eating guidelines you'll find on MyPyramid.gov (pages 24–25), you'll easily get the forty essential nutrients your body needs for peak performance and well-being, while at the same time managing your weight. Like a smart shopper who gets the best value for her money, following the guidelines of MyPyramid will give your body the most vitamins, minerals, protein and other nutrients with the fewest calories. But that's not all: Almost every day, new nutrition research emerges to support the fact that eating a healthful diet can bring you other amazing benefits.

YOU COULD FEEL MORE SUSTAINED ENERGY People who follow a healthful eating plan may find that they don't feel as many peaks and valleys of energy as they do when they eat unhealthfully. When you fuel your body using the MyPyramid recommendations, you'll give your body a combination of carbohydrates for quick energy, protein to sustain your body and a little fat for long-term energy. In short, your body's energy level will feel more in balance all day long. However, without this combination of nutrients, your blood sugar and corresponding energy level may behave like a roller-coaster ride. During a drop in energy, your brain may be more likely to guide you to reach for foods that will quickly raise your energy level, only to have it plunge again later.

YOU COULD LIVE A MORE POSITIVE LIFE With the sustained energy levels you could begin to feel while you're enjoying a more healthful eating plan, you may be more likely to break free from what some weight-management experts refer to as a "cycle of inactivity." As pounds start to drop, the exercise that helps promote weight management (pages 36–41) could well begin to feel more possible, even pleasurable, marking the beginning of a new, positive, more active cycle in your life.

YOU COULD REDUCE YOUR RISK FACTORS FOR DISEASE Medical studies have shown that direct correlations exist between eating a healthful diet and a greater likelihood of wellness. If you follow the guidelines in MyPyramid—eating a diet abounding in plant-based foods and with limited saturated fats and sodium—you could decrease what medical science has found to be risk factors for a wide range of diseases including various forms of cancer, gastrointestinal illnesses and cardiovascular disease.

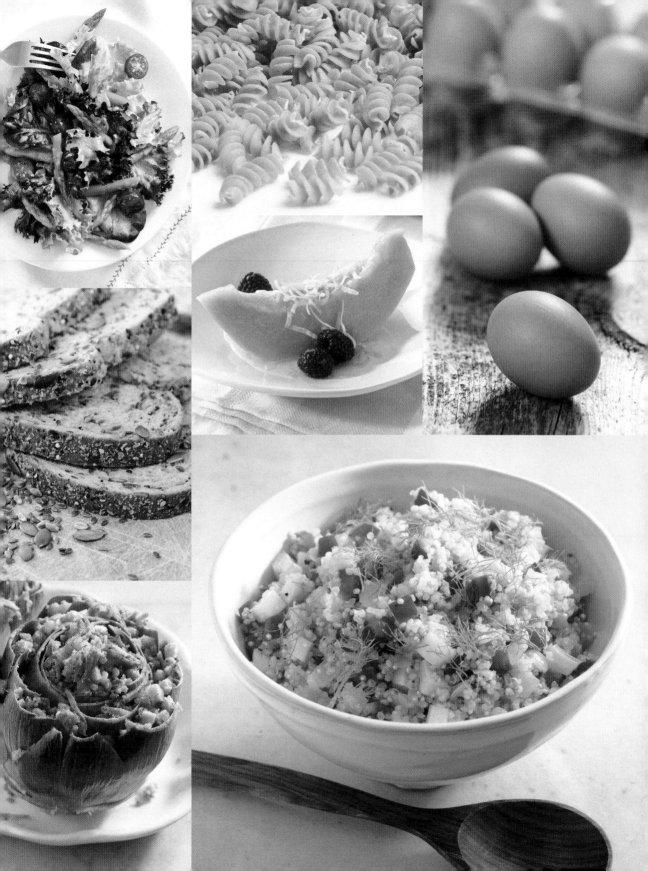

The Key to Managing Your Hunger

Finding delicious ways to feel comfortably full or satisfied is an important tool for weight management. Simply put, the greater the feeling of satiety you get from food, the less you'll eat. All kinds of healthful foods can give you satiety, including those that boast high amounts of fiber, protein, water, good fats, hot spices and intense flavors. Compare those suggested here to the categories on MyPyramid (pages 24–25) and notice that high-satiety foods are also some of the healthiest.

FIBER Fiber keeps you feeling full longer by slowing the movement of food through your digestive system. It also helps reduce the risk of heart disease and cancer, while helping to promote digestive health. Many cereals, including most **Special K®** cereals (apart from **Special K** Original cereal) are good sources of fiber, and many contain whole grains. Other sources of fiber include such whole-grain foods as whole-grain breads, brown rice, whole-wheat pasta and bulgur; vegetables, including sweet potatoes, spinach, green peas, cooked cabbage and hard-shelled squash; fruits with edible skins or seeds, such as apples, pears, raspberries and figs; and beans and lentils, which are also sources of protein.

PROTEIN Digested slowly, protein helps you avoid hunger pangs. Get protein from such sources as nonfat milk, **Special K** foods with protein; eggs or egg products; lean meats, poultry or seafood; and legumes.

WATER-DENSE FOODS Many studies have found that foods that are higher in water volume and correspondingly lower in calories—such as vegetables, fruits, cooked oatmeal and brothy soups—take a long time to eat, so you feel satisfied. And water bound to these foods stays in your system for a long time, keeping your hunger at bay.

FATS AND OILS Fats and oils are calorie dense, but if you eat them in small portions, they can deliver loads of satisfaction. For example, try a little aged blue cheese over salad or whole-grain pasta or served with fresh fruit; or use 1 teaspoon of extra-virgin olive oil as part of salad dressings or for light sautéing.

HOT SPICES AND INTENSE FLAVORS Spices bring satisfaction by waking up your taste buds. People tend to eat spicy foods very slowly, so they also feel satisfied with less. Full-flavored foods also encourage slow savoring. The recipes in this book (pages 65–231) have been developed to offer vivid tastes that will leave you feeling more satisfied with sensible-sized portions.

CALORIE Q & A

Calories is the buzzword on many weight-management plans, but their use and importance are often misunderstood. The following answers to some of the most common questions about calories can help you achieve your own weight-management victory.

What are calories?

A: Calories are measurement units for energy—both the energy food and drink provide, and the energy our bodies use.

Where does the idea of calories come from?

A: The measurement was originally developed to measure heat in laboratory studies (one calorie equals the amount of energy it takes to raise the temperature of 1 gram of water by 1° Celsius). Calories used to measure the energy provided by food or burned off through exercise are technically "kilocalories," one thousand times greater than the laboratory measurement. However, when talking about food and exercise, one calorie and one kilocalorie are identical.

How do calories relate to weight management?

A: Take in more calories than your body needs, and you'll gain weight. Take in fewer and burn them up more through regular exercise, and you'll lose weight.

How many calories can I eat in a day?

A: The average woman needs 1,500 to 2,000 calories daily to maintain a healthy weight. To lose one pound of body weight, you need to burn 3,500 calories more than you take in.

Must I really count calories?

A: Not necessarily. If you observe daily serving guidelines for each of the food groups suggested in MyPyramid (pages 24–25), learn portion control and eat only until you feel comfortably satisfied (page 31), you'll take in the right amount of calories you need without counting.

How do I keep track of my weight-management goals?

A: Counting calories helps some people feel in control. If counting works for you, consult a printed calorie guide, or search the Internet for one of the many online sources. Whether you are a calorie counter or not, you can keep track of your daily calorie intake or other weight management goals by recording them in the journal pages on pages 232–233.

Change Your Food Behavior

We tend to learn our attitudes toward food and the ways in which we eat it starting in childhood. As much as successful weight management depends upon making the right choices in *what* you eat, it also depends upon *how* you eat. The good news is that you can change your behavior relating to food. The key is to develop the habit of stopping and wondering *why* you eat the way you do and then learning to eat more mindfully, which employs three simple strategies: know your food personality; slow down and savor; and practice portion control.

> *"Most of us don't overeat because we're hungry," observes eating behavior expert and author Brian Wansink, Ph.D., former executive director of the USDA's Center for Nutrition Policy and Promotion. At his web site www.MindlessEating.org, Wansink observes that all sorts of other cues can cause us to want to eat, including the influence of the people around us, images we see in media, and the aromas, sights and sounds of food we encounter in our everyday lives.*

KNOW YOUR FOOD PERSONALITY One good way to start learning mindful eating is to think about what kind of eater you are. What aspects of your daily life influence how you eat? Does one of these scenarios sound familiar?

- Too often, your food choices depend on what your children eat. Your food pleasures are those in which you indulge yourself after you put the kids to bed.

- Many of your eating decisions depend on what's offered at hotel restaurants or airport cafes. Snacks from the mini bar are common meal replacements.

- You don't make time for meals until you notice you're starving. Meals of vending-machine food or takeout at your desk are frequent.

- You eat meals mindlessly between remote-control or mouse clicks or while chatting with friends on your computer or smartphone.

As you can see from the examples above, your circumstances can lead to eating behaviors that don't help you maintain your weight. Once you understand what kind of eater you are—whether you are a busy mom, business traveler, workaholic or multitasker—you can plan your meals mindfully and set yourself up for success.

SLOW DOWN AND SAVOR Many scientific studies have shown that it takes a while after you start eating before your brain's appetite-control center recognizes that your hunger has been satisfied. So, the more slowly you eat, the less food you'll need to feel full. Here are some pleasurable ways to slow down and eat more mindfully: Turn off the television. Set an attractive table. Then, use all your senses to enjoy your meal slowly and fully. See how beautiful the food looks. Breathe in and enjoy its aromas. Finally, take a small bite. Chew the food slowly, at least 20 times. Put down your cutlery. Swallow and sip some water before taking your next small bite. After 20 minutes, ask yourself: Do I still feel hungry? If the answer is no, stop eating. Remember: It's *okay* not to finish everything on your plate!

PRACTICE PORTION CONTROL Recommended portion sizes for healthful meals (see below) can look small to modern eyes. One reason is that the average portion sizes have grown larger to fill our ever-larger dinner plates. Half a century ago, many dinner plates were only 9 inches in diameter. Today, many are 12 inches and can hold about 75 percent more food than in decades past. Instead of feeling deprived, use a salad plate instead of a dinner plate and fill it up. Using your eyes to trick your brain, a plateful of food will look and feel as satisfying as a full-size dinner plate. If you don't already own small dinner plates, look for them in kitchenware or department stores.

Guide to portion sizes

Instead of carrying a food scale or measuring cup everywhere you go, compare foods to everyday objects. It's easy to recognize the right portion sizes.

- One serving of pancake or waffle is equal in diameter to a compact disk
- A ½-cup serving of fruits or vegetables is about the size of a tennis ball
- A ¼-cup serving of dried fruit or nuts is about the size of a golf ball
- A 3-ounce serving of fish fillet is about the size of a checkbook
- A 3-ounce serving of poultry or meat is equal to a deck of cards
- One medium baked potato is about the size of a computer mouse
- A 1-ounce serving of cheese is about the size of a 1 x 1 x 1-inch cube

The Importance of Snacking

Hunger pangs between meals are signals that we need some food and the energy it provides. Food cravings, too, can often have logical biochemical reasons. Chocolate, for example, contains compounds that increase the release of endorphins into your bloodstream, which help relieve stress and increase calmness—your body might "crave" the feeling created by eating chocolate as much as it does the flavor and the energy boost that it provides.

In short, you need snacks, so there's no need to deprive yourself. In fact, snacking may help you manage your weight more easily. That being said, successful weight management depends on knowing when to eat snacks, choosing and enjoying the right kinds of snacks and eating them in the right amounts. Try these strategies to help make healthful, satisfying snacking part of your daily life.

TIME AND PLAN YOUR SNACKS If you plan ahead, you are less likely to eat snacks you'll regret later. Snack sensibly, and you'll feel ready for your next scheduled mealtime and will be less likely to overeat. Staying on track with snacks and mealtimes is important: Your body gets used to being fed at certain times, and keeping a routine keeps your metabolism humming right along. But if you snack too close to mealtime, you might decide to skip or delay the meal, which could lead to feeling super-hungry and overeating later. (If you have diabetes, it's especially important to eat at the same time and in similar amounts daily, to help avoid dramatic swings in blood-sugar level.) Here are some tips for snacking that will help keep you on track:

- Enjoy daytime snacks two to three hours before a meal
- Pre-pack snacks in plastic bags or containers to take with you during a busy day
- Gather some healthful **Special K®** snacks to take along if you'll be out
- Pay attention to portion size
- If you tend to get hungry before bedtime, consider adding a small, sensible late-evening snack such as a serving of your favorite **Special K** cereal or snack food
- Savor your snacks slowly, as you would a meal

USE SNACKS TO FILL IN THE GAPS Snacking provides key opportunities to help you get in all the different kinds of foods you need for nutritional balance. For example, do you find it difficult to get in MyPyramid's suggested 3 cups per day of milk products? Then try a dairy snack. Not getting enough fruits and vegetables? Try a small apple or a handful of baby carrots.

DON'T GO OVERBOARD Just as when you are eating meals, try to avoid overindulging when snacking. Enjoy sensibly sized portions, and keep track of snacks in your food journal (pages 232–233). If you're counting daily calories, be sure to include snacks in your calorie totals. That doesn't mean that you can't have a snack that's a little more indulgent from time to time. Knowing that you don't need to deprive yourself may sometimes make it easier to feel satisfied with a smaller serving that still fits within your daily goals.

AVOID THE MUNCHIES If your attention is drawn elsewhere, it's hard to slow down and enjoy a snack to the point of savoring it. So be careful that your snack time doesn't overlap with watching TV, catching up on emails or phone calls or when working on a stressful deadline. Of course, at times you will be distracted and still need a snack. In such cases, make sure your snack is pre-portioned, and choose something sensible and healthful that takes a long time to eat.

Snacks that pack a punch

Snacks that include both carbohydrates and protein will provide quick and sustained energy to help hold hunger at bay until your next meal. Try sensibly sized portions of nutrient-rich options such as:

- **Special K®** crackers and hummus
- Sliced pear or apple with low-fat cheese
- Yogurt-and-fruit smoothie
- Whole wheat pita bread half with water-packed canned tuna
- Small quesadilla with melted low-fat cheese
- **Special K** cereal or snack bar and nonfat milk

Season Your Meals with Variety

We've all heard the saying that variety is the spice of life. Whether you cook at home or enjoy meals out, if you aim for livelier variety, you'll be more satisfied with portions of a sensible size, feel more in control and truly enjoy what you eat.

MIX UP YOUR INGREDIENTS Refer regularly to MyPyramid (pages 24–25) to make sure you get your daily servings from all food groups. Beyond that, try seeking out exciting new kinds of fruits and vegetables, grains and seafood you haven't tried before. Or, bring excitement to your meals by combining different taste sensations. For example, mix sweet (fresh or dried fruit); salty (capers, olives, anchovies or Parmesan cheese); bitter (dark greens like arugula, escarole or kale); and sour (citrus, grapes, vinegar, yogurt) in complementary portions.

In 1908, Japanese research chemist Dr. Kikunae Ikeda identified a fifth taste sensation, called umami. Described as "deep," "rich," "meaty," or "satisfying," umami has been found to help produce a feeling of satiety. It is present in foods like tomatoes, dark mushrooms, beef, pork, chicken, Parmesan and blue cheeses, and many types of fish and shellfish.

EXPLORE NEW CUISINES The recipes in this book offer tastes from around the globe. Try dining out with different cuisines as well. Many ethnic restaurants include healthful, low-fat options—and most, if you ask, will prepare dishes with little oil or with sauce or dressing on the side.

SEASON WITH IMAGINATION Seasonings don't mean just salt and pepper. Herbs, spices and other aromatic ingredients make every bite worth savoring and are virtually calorie free. When you cook, aim to include more herbs and spices, adjusting quantities as you grow more confident. Soon you'll be a seasoning expert.

CONTRAST COLORS AND TEXTURES As the old saying goes, you eat with your eyes first. Enliven meals with beautiful, nutrient-packed ingredients: orange sweet potatoes, purple and yellow beets, red tomatoes and pomegranates, green okra, yellow sweet corn, orange apricots and peaches, indigo blueberries, tan mushrooms, brown wild rice, ivory jicama. Varied textures—soft, creamy, chewy, crisp, crunchy—enhance pleasure, too, helping you slow down to savor every bite.

DEALING WITH DINING OUT

Sticking to your weight-management goals can be tricky when you are away from home. Try these clever strategies to help you stay on track when eating in restaurants, when you are on vacation or at parties and celebrations.

In restaurants

- Review menus online in advance to focus on your smartest options

- Say a polite "no, thank you" when the server offers you bread

- Instead of ordering an appetizer and main course, order two appetizers; or, split a main dish with someone else

- Before you even start eating, pay attention to what a proper portion size would be (page 31), and ask your server to wrap up the rest for you

- If dessert is irresistible, order just one for the table to share

On vacation

- Read the menus that many cafés and restaurants post outside, focusing on healthful options

- Take breakfast from a hotel buffet, choosing sensible portions of healthful foods including fruit, whole grains, nonfat or low-fat dairy, lean meats and eggs cooked with little or no fat

- Visit local markets for healthful options to keep in your room for breakfast or lunch or to carry with you for picnic meals or as snacks

- Aim to walk as much as possible—it's a great way to burn calories while sightseeing

At parties

- To compensate for temptations, plan to eat fewer calories than usual a day or two before and after the event

- To help you choose more wisely, politely question the hosts about the menu in advance

- If time allows, add 10 to 15 minutes to your daily exercise routine

- Before you leave for a party, eat a healthful snack (pages 32–33)

- At the party, drink lots of still or sparkling water, adding a wedge of lemon or lime if you like; this will help keep you feeling full and refreshed

- To help you keep your health-conscious wits about you, limit your intake of beverages containing alcohol; try a wine spritzer, mixing white wine and sparkling water

- After selecting food from a buffet, step away from the table to help avoid absent-minded munching

Exercise for Weight Management

Whether you've embarked on **The Special K Challenge**™ or have moved beyond that kick-start phase, exercise plays an essential role in helping you achieve your weight-management goal. By itself, eating wisely may help you lose pounds and inches, but combining it with regular, enjoyable exercise increases the odds that you'll continue to trim down while you maintain high energy and vibrant health.

> *Guidelines issued in 2007 by the American Heart Association and the American College of Sports Medicine suggest that "60 to 90 minutes of physical activity may be necessary" most days for significant weight loss.*

Whether you exercise just 30 minutes per day (the minimum recommended by MyPyramid, pages 24–25) or the more ambitious 60–90 minutes suggested by the American Heart Association (above), the time you spend engaging in physical activity can be a pleasure. If you wish, you can break up the activity into 10-minute segments throughout the day, including walking briskly, dancing vigorously to music, or doing strenuous housework or gardening as well as spending time at the gym. But in order for an exercise program to be sustainable, it should also be fun. You can learn to make it that way—and eliminate the feeling of *work* from your workouts—with the help of the information on the following pages.

Let's begin by understanding the different general categories of exercise: stretching (or flexibility), cardio training (aerobic exercise) and strength training (resistance). Each plays its own role in contributing to your well-being. Remember: *Always check with your doctor before starting any exercise program*. It's also a good idea to book a session with a fitness trainer to make sure you're exercising safely and effectively.

STRETCHING Slow, relaxed, gentle stretches of the muscles in your neck, shoulders, arms and hands; back, waist and hips; legs, ankles and feet—this may be the most overlooked kind of exercise. Before and after you perform cardio- or strength-training exercises, aim to stretch for five to seven minutes, breathing slowly and naturally. Stretching will prepare your body for the exertion to come by raising your heart rate, loosening muscles and joints, increasing blood flow to your muscles and helping you avoid injury.

Check with your health club or search online for a stretching routine that works for you. You can stretch while standing, lying down on a mat or leaning against a wall—whatever works best for you. Some prefer to use props to aid in stretching, such as elastic cords or large inflatable exercise balls.

CARDIO TRAINING Regular aerobic activity that gets your heart and lungs working hard enough to make you break a sweat is essential. Nothing else burns as many calories: from 170 calories for 30 minutes of brisk walking (for someone weighing 150 pounds) to twice that many for 30 minutes of step aerobics. Besides those two exercises, you have so many more options. Choose something that you really enjoy, such as running, bicycling, cross-country skiing, indoor elliptical or treadmill or stair-climber machines, swimming, inline skating, kick boxing, jumping rope, soccer, basketball and vigorous dancing; all of these activities are considered aerobic. But how can you tell if your heart rate is high enough to gain the most benefit?

- First, calculate your maximum heart rate by subtracting your age from 220. For example, a 35-year-old's maximum heart rate would be 185 beats per minute (220 − 35 = 185).

- Next, check your pulse at your wrist, or at your neck just below the jaw, counting the number of beats that occur in 15 seconds; then, multiply by 4 to calculate your heart rate per minute.

- Finally, increase or decrease your activity as needed with the aim of reaching 75 to 80 percent of your maximum heart rate. The 35-year-old in the example above should strive for a heart rate no higher than 148 beats per minute (185 x 0.8 = 148).

STRENGTH TRAINING Even when you are resting, your muscle tissue burns calories more quickly than fat tissue. So, the higher your body's percentage of muscle, the more calories you'll burn all day. Strength training involves so-called "resistance" exercises in which you exert specific muscles, usually by lifting or pulling weights. Consult with a trainer to find the best routine for you and the safe, right way to do it, aiming for at least two nonconsecutive days a week, including exercises for your arms, chest, shoulders, back, abdomen, hips and upper and lower legs. Don't worry that you might "bulk up." In general, using lighter weights and higher numbers of repetitions tones and subtly builds muscles, giving you a sleeker look.

Mix Up Your Exercise Routine

Just as variety can spice up your healthful eating plan, so too can varying your exercise keep you on track on your personal weight-management journey. The key to success is to think about what kind of physical activities you really enjoy, and find ways to incorporate those activities into your daily and weekly life as much as possible.

Of course, that doesn't mean you have to search continually for new experiences, either. Some people find a form of exercise they truly love—whether it's swimming or running, dancing or fencing—and dedicate themselves to doing it as often as possible.

But many of us thrive on new experiences, just like we enjoy different tastes on our plates. If you are a variety-is-the-spice-of-life kind of person, start thinking about your exercise options as a fabulous buffet full of choices—but this time, it's a buffet you can feel free to sample from as much as you like. Mixing up your routines may actually help you get more out of your exercise, too:

Some studies have shown that if you do the same kind of exercises day after day, week after week, your body and muscles could get so habituated to the routine and so efficient at performing it that they reach a plateau at which you may no longer get maximum benefit from doing them.

EMBRACE CHANGE Experts recommend changing the exercise from time to time—whether finding another form of cardio training that you find enjoyable or using a different kind of weight machine to target the same muscles. By doing so, you may be targeting different parts of the same muscle groups, which could help you tone even more. At the same time, you could find that you're enjoying a fresh new approach to exercise that will help keep you engaged.

BE KIND TO YOURSELF Too many people slack off on their commitment to regular exercise because they have an all-or-nothing mentality. If you can't manage a daily 60-to-90-minute session at the health club, that doesn't mean you have failed. Remember: You don't have to accomplish your daily exercise all at once. If it works better for you and your lifestyle, break up your exercise into smaller, more manageable parts, aiming for a minimum of 30 minutes of activity and a blend of stretching, cardio training and strength building.

EVERY LITTLE BIT COUNTS

Think of ways you can squeeze in ten-minute parcels of activity here and there as part of your routines, and your daily exercise time will add up before you know it. Try these ideas to start, and jot down in your journal new healthy habits to remind yourself to keep moving.

Park farther or exit earlier Pick a spot at the farthest end of the parking lot from your office or other destination. Or, if you travel by bus or subway, get off one stop sooner. Those extra daily steps add up.

Swear off the elevator If you can, take the stairs instead of the elevator. Even just going down the stairs means more calories are burned.

Leave your desk If you have a desk job, make a point to move every hour, whether to personally deliver a message to someone in another office or just to circle the floor or building. You'll break up the monotony of your workday, maybe build new friendships with coworkers, and definitely add some fitness to your 9-to-5.

Get off the couch At home, pop in an exercise DVD or turn up your favorite tunes and dance around. Re-create a routine from your favorite exercise class. Climb the stairs a few times or take a brisk stroll around the block.

Make prime time your time Instead of taking a seat on the sofa or relaxing in bed while you watch TV, catch up on your favorite shows *and* your fitness routine at the same time. Find a spot on the floor and concentrate on strength training during those shows. During a commercial break, take your heart rate up a notch with sets of jumping jacks, lunges, and push-ups.

Hop to it Jumping rope provides a great full-body workout—remember how much fun it was when you were a kid? If the gym dues strain your finances, pick up a rope and start hopping instead.

Make your exercise playful Remember how much fun it was to play active games when you were a kid? Consider joining your children, or organizing your grown-up friends, for a trip to the park to jump rope, play tennis or badminton, kick around a soccer ball, or another activity that you love. Even flying a kite can add some movement to your day.

Walk the dog Your four-legged friend could become your best exercise companion. Instead of leaving your pet to run around the back yard by itself, hook up the leash and head out into the neighborhood for lively morning and evening strolls that could do both of you a world of good.

Stick to Your Exercise Goals

Exercising four or five days a week can help make a noticeable contribution to your weight-management goals. But real victory, of course, comes with sticking to it.

The key to success is finding ways to stay on track with your exercise plans. Sure, work or school commitments, family demands or simply our social lives can sometimes compete with exercise time. But there is a simple way to increase the likelihood that you'll meet your goals: Make them realistic and achievable.

A research study conducted in 2005 by the American College of Sports Medicine gave two separate randomly assigned groups of inactive adults pedometers to wear, with the goal of increasing how many steps they took daily. One group was asked to add 2,500 steps to a daily baseline of 5,510 steps. A second group was given the more difficult goal of taking 10,000 steps per day. After eight weeks, 42.3 percent of the former group succeeded an average of four days a week. By contrast, only 15.4 percent of the latter group succeeded in the same amount of time.

The study referred to above illustrates that setting realistic goals for your weight-management plan may give a higher rate of success. Along with variety in your exercise routine (pages 38–39), be sure you are being realistic when you plan it. The following tips are also helpful:

MAKE IT FUN Finding physical activities that you enjoy—and can stick to—means they might evolve into hobbies, and increase your chance of continuing them for the long term. To increase your odds of doing them, seek out people you know who might share these activities with you—such as a significant other, friend, or coworker—and invite them to join you on a regular, even-scheduled basis.

JOIN IN Some people like or need to exercise alone, but many find it more fun to exercise with a group. Joining a health club with a range of facilities that appeal to you could be an answer to keeping your routine varied and fun. Most offer a variety of group exercise classes free to members. But it doesn't necessarily have to be an exclusive or expensive club. Investigate reasonably priced options available in your area, including YMCAs, cultural centers and other community organizations. Many neighborhoods have running and walking clubs as well as organizations that feature all kinds of other physical activities. Ask your friends and neighbors and check local publications or online for opportunities near you.

GET EXPERT HELP Whatever you decide to do, be sure to seek guidance from a certified trainer or coach who can make sure you're exercising correctly and safely and will gain the maximum benefits. Most health clubs or gyms have experts on hand who can lead you through new exercise programs. As you progress, check in with a trainer on a regular basis or when you want to change your routine. If you exercise at home, follow a reputable online video or DVD program to help stay on track.

BEWARE OF PITFALLS When you find a realistic exercise plan you enjoy, watch out for a phenomenon some experts call "compensation." This happens when, after a good workout, people reward themselves with calorie-laden goodies that give their tired, hungry bodies bursts of energy; or when, after strenuous exercise, your tiredness becomes an excuse to take it easy the rest of the day.

Tips to avoid compensation

An occasional indulgence won't derail your journey—as long as such self-rewards don't become a habit. Try these tips to help you avoid "compensation" and help you stay on track:

- Write down your healthful eating plan in your daily calendar so that it is always with you to ward off temptations
- Eat a healthful meal or snack 30 minutes to an hour before you exercise to help stave off hunger pangs during your workout
- Have a healthful snack on hand (pages 32–33) to enjoy after your workout
- Weave more activity into the fabric of your daily life (pages 38–39) so you'll be less inclined to take it easy
- Share your weight-management goals with your exercise buddy and enlist her help in achieving them

Succeed through Mind and Spirit

At this point, you've given yourself a kick-start with **The Special K Challenge**™ (pages 13–19). You understand the basics of a healthful, varied, and delicious eating plan (pages 24–35). And you know how important it is to exercise regularly (pages 36–41). But just as food and exercise work together to help you manage your weight, there's still another key to success: the way you *think* and *feel*.

That doesn't mean you can just "think yourself" to a healthier weight. Or that meditation or relaxation alone can make it happen. But taking steps, whatever they might be, to relax and feel more positive about yourself and your goals can definitely help. Remember, though, that no two people are alike. Just as your favorite healthful foods or preferred exercise may differ from someone else's, so may the mind and spirit approach that works best for you. The way you think and feel may help support your efforts to manage your weight. Try these ideas, or list others that work for you in your weight-management journal so you can easily remember them.

SET MEASURABLE GOALS One of the best ways to stay positive during your journey is to set goals that are not only realistic, but also measurable. Include everything from how much weight you'd like to lose, such as "I'll drop four or five pounds in a month"; to positive steps you can take, like "I'll try at least one new healthful recipe per week this month"; to regular weight-management behaviors, like "I'll use measuring cups and a kitchen scale when cooking to double-check portion sizes"; or "I'll weigh myself weekly" (page 53). Sticking to such simple goals will make it easier—and more rewarding—for you to measure your progress.

USE SLEEP TO KEEP YOU ON TRACK Before you go to bed, write down your achievements and your goals, and imagine the vibrant, energetic and healthy self you're in the process of becoming. Before you nod off, relax your body, quiet your mind, and consider what you would like to dream about tonight that will be in line with your program. Aim to get seven to eight hours of sleep every night, which will help combat stress and keep your mind sharp and able to make smart decisions. When you awake the next morning, write down any victorious dreams you can remember and how you feel about them. Take some time while your mind is still relaxed to write down your positive thoughts and offer yourself words of encouragement for the new day to come.

VISUALIZE SUCCESS Imagine how you will look and feel when your reach your weight-management goal and find a visual cue to inspire you. Maybe you're aiming to look and feel like a time in your past when you felt you were your best self? Tape a picture of yourself at your best to the bathroom mirror and let it inspire you anew every day. Or maybe there's an inspirational saying or verse that gives you a feeling of peace and strength. Attach it to your refrigerator or pantry door to help you keep your mind on your goals every time you prepare a meal or reach for a snack. Another idea is to put a framed a photograph of you with your loved ones to serve as a good reminder of why you want to manage your weight and live a longer, more active life.

HARNESS THE POWER OF THE MIND Some people find that psychology and talk therapy may help them manage their weight. Sometimes, weight-management efforts can be complicated by other personal issues from the past. Therapy can help you address them and find new understanding to help you stick to your goals.

In a study conducted at Huddinge University Hospital in Stockholm, Sweden, and published in March 2005 in the journal Eating and Weight Disorders, *patients in a ten-week weight-loss program that included cognitive therapy not only lost weight, but 18 months later, had kept it off. Some subjects had lost even more weight. Meanwhile, a control group without therapy actually gained weight.*

If private therapy is not within your means or not something with which you feel comfortable, look for individual or group support at a community center, place of worship or local medical school that could be more affordable or approachable.

TRY AN ALTERNATIVE THERAPY Some people find hypnosis to be a valuable tool in succeeding on a weight-management plan. Look online for a licensed and certified hypnotherapist or hypnotherapy center in your community.

DON'T GO IT ALONE Consider the possibility that you will find it even easier to achieve your weight-management goals with the help of other people who are on the same journey. There are many great, easy ways to get the help and support you need and deserve (pages 44–45).

Enlist the Support of Others

Sure, successful weight management requires you to make a personal commitment. But you may find that once you join forces with others, the weight-management journey you're setting out on can be not only a more enjoyable experience—and an opportunity to make great new friends—but also a chance to see yourself more positively through the eyes of others.

In a Gallup Poll Panel study released in 2005, 56 percent of American women thought they were "at least somewhat overweight." Time and again, surveys and studies show that a majority of women have negative body images centered on weighing too much.

By telling people you know about the commitment you've made to weight management, or by joining others who are managing their weight, you will enjoy one of the most useful assets imaginable: support. And today more than ever, there are so many ways for you to get that support. Here are just a few of the options:

FORM A CLUB Once you tell friends or people you know from your school, parents' group, health club, place of worship or somewhere else you frequent and feel secure, you'll probably find that other people start opening up to you about their weight-management goals. It's a small step from there to organizing a regular weekly meeting where everybody weighs in; shares victories and setbacks; swaps healthful recipes, ideas and inspirations; and maybe even teams up as exercise partners.

ENROLL IN A GROUP There are many organizations, some nonprofit and others for-profit businesses, that function as support groups for people who want to make a commitment to weight management. Choose a group that sounds right for you and works with your schedule and budget. Find out which program is best for you by asking a trusted friend or by reading about the options online.

ASK A BUDDY Organized clubs or groups aren't for everybody. If you prefer, consider asking a friend to be your weight-management buddy. Having just one other person ready to cheer you on and be there for support can make a difference. And you might discover that you gain just as much strength yourself by being a source of strength for someone else.

JOIN AN ONLINE COMMUNITY If meeting in person is not your cup of tea, there are also online groups that lend good support "virtually." A brief Internet search will help you uncover many Web sites offering weight-management support. For example, you'll find useful, supportive resources at www.SpecialK.com, where experts in such fields as nutrition, health, cooking, exercise and fashion—and many thousands of people just like you who have already taken **The Special K Challenge**™—share a wealth of information, inspiration and advice.

Add an incentive

Some people find that incentives encourage them to stay on track even more. Try one of the following suggestions, or let them inspire your own ideas to help you reach your weight-management goals.

Reward yourself Set a milestone for pounds or inches lost, and then promise yourself—or have a loved one promise you—some sort of reward when you reach it. Ideas include a charm for your bracelet, a massage at a nearby spa, or a new outfit.

Start a pool Challenge your weight-management buddy or club members to put up a small amount of money. The first one to reach an agreed-upon (sensible) milestone wins the pot.

Put your "pounds" on display Choose some kind of small, inexpensive object you find beautiful—it could be a seashell, a paperweight, a pretty pair of earrings—to represent a regular milestone such as five or ten pounds lost. Buy one every time you achieve that goal and put it on display, lining them up on a shelf or jewelry stand to remind you of all the personal victories you've achieved.

Think big For a major milestone, treat yourself to something big like a weekend getaway or a vacation to an exotic destination where you can wear a new swimsuit.

Reduce Stress

Do you know people who reach for their favorite comfort food or junk food when they feel stressed out? Do you count yourself among them? You aren't alone.

According to a 2006 survey of American eating habits published by the Pew Research Center, "there is a correlation between stress and eating." Among survey respondents who described themselves as frequently stressed, 21 percent said they overate often, and 25 percent said they ate too much junk food too often. Those percentages were dramatically lower for people who said that they rarely or never felt stressed.

Along with healthful eating and regular exercise, reducing stress is an important part of successful weight management. All kinds of factors can create stress. Fortunately, proven strategies can significantly reduce, if not eliminate, stress. Choose one that feels right and works best for you.

- Eat healthful, well-balanced meals (pages 24–35); cut down on sugar, caffeine and alcohol; exercise regularly (pages 36–41); and get enough sleep.

- Avoid stressful people, heated conversation topics, and sensationalist news. Learn to say "no" to tasks that you find stressful and that you don't really need to do.

- If a situation stresses you, talk with other people involved and find a way to make things more calm and pleasant for everyone. If you always feel rushed or like you are falling behind, look for ways to rearrange your schedule.

- If you're a perfectionist, realize that few things need to be perfect. Think back to past situations that may have caused you stress but came out okay. Remind yourself that the stressful situations you're dealing with today will probably end up fine.

- However busy you are, make time for activities that bring you pleasure. Try to include regular activities that have the specific goal of relaxation (see opposite page).

- If things still feel too stressful, consider speaking with your doctor, counselor or spiritual advisor. Some people find that prayer or meditation helps them eliminate stress and manage their weight.

RELAXATION TECHNIQUES

Many different techniques can help reduce stress. Whatever you try, first find out as much as you can about it from expert sources to make sure you practice it safely and effectively. When seeking outside help, work only with trained, certified and reputable professionals.

Acupuncture or acupressure When practiced by a trained and certified professional, this process of stimulating certain points on the body using fine needles or the application of fingertip pressure has been found to reduce stress.

Deep breathing Simply inhaling and exhaling in the right way can bring quick relief at stressful moments. Sit upright in a chair, close your eyes and take a series of deep breaths, starting deep in your abdomen, slowly but comfortably breathing in through your nose and then out from your mouth.

Deep relaxation Whether guided by a trained hypnotherapist (page 43), or self-guided through techniques that you can learn easily, this deep-relaxation method not only helps to ease stress, but can also reinforce positive habits and self-images.

Massage A spa session can help release stress where your body stores it, in stiff and knotted muscles.

Meditation and prayer Quiet reflection and concentration on a restful, soothing word, image or verse is one way to distance yourself from the world's cares.

Muscle relaxation Combined with deep breathing while lying down with the eyes closed, this process of briefly tensing and slowly releasing your muscles—starting at the feet and gradually working up to the face—provides relief for many people.

Positive visualization Similar to hypnosis and meditation, this guided or self-induced technique can help you relax deeply while you imagine restful scenes and positive images. Close your eyes, breathe slowly and deeply, and picture your best self.

Reflexology In this ancient Chinese therapeutic technique, a trained professional applies pressure to specific spots on the feet or hands to affect other parts of the body. Some studies have found that reflexology can help reduce stress.

Yoga Combining gentle movements, poses and stretches with slow, deep breathing, this ancient eastern practice reduces stress for many people, especially when carefully guided in a class or by a private yoga teacher.

How to Deal with Temptations

The people who manage their weight most successfully have learned how to use common sense when dealing with cravings. Rather than resisting temptations with an iron will or giving in completely, it's a matter of recognizing cravings for what they are and learning to control them sensibly.

When you deal with temptations in sensible ways, you'll feel more positive about yourself, more powerful and more in control. Following are some sound tips to help you stave off cravings and stay on track.

BECOME A MORE SAVVY CONSUMER Arming yourself with information will make it more likely that you'll make sensible food purchases. To help you make smarter choices, understand what food package labels really mean and how to use them. According to U.S. federal guidelines, "calorie-free" foods are fewer than five calories per serving; "low-calorie" foods are fewer than 40 calories per serving; "light" or "lite" foods contain a third fewer calories or 50 percent less fat than a standard serving size of the same food in its regular form. Turn to page 55 for more information on Nutrition Facts panels on packaged foods and how to use them.

BE THE GATEKEEPER In most households, one person is the main grocery shopper. If it's you, resist buying the less-than-healthful treats enjoyed by the others in the household. If something you crave is not in your home, it can't tempt you as easily. Your family members will forgive you—and they can and will get used to eating more fruits, vegetables, whole grains and low-fat or nonfat dairy products, giving their health a boost as well as yours. If you are not the gatekeeper, be sure to give the shopper a list of healthful foods you need to stay on track.

PRESS THE PAUSE BUTTON One simple trick for dealing with temptations or cravings is to imagine pressing a "pause button" in your head. As you would when watching a movie, "press" that pause button when you want to interrupt your usual behavior, such as indulging in a regular craving. Use that pause to ask yourself, "Why do I have this craving right now?" Has something upset or worried you and you're looking for the comfort a favorite food can offer? Do you habitually crave something in a certain situation, like popcorn at the movies or ice cream after a dinner of Chinese food? This brief interruption helps you to make a conscious decision to substitute a healthier choice. Maybe you'll reach for a nutritious snack. Perhaps you'll choose a small popcorn instead of a large. Maybe you'll opt for a single scoop of fat-free sorbet instead of super-premium ice cream. Or maybe that pause will give you the time you need to realize that you aren't really hungry at all.

DO SOMETHING OTHER THAN EATING If you find that stress triggers bouts of eating, consider doing something else instead. Other activities can reduce stress far more effectively than food. For example, listen to music you love or pick up a favorite instrument. Watch a video on the Internet that always makes you laugh. Talk to a supportive friend or family member (pages 44–45). Get in 10 minutes of exercise (pages 36–37). Or write about your craving and feelings in your weight-management journal (pages 52–53, 232–233).

GIVE IN—JUST A LITTLE You can also allow yourself a small amount of what you crave. Thinking of food as "forbidden" may cause you to crave it even more. Unless you are avoiding something for specific medical reasons, tell yourself you can have a small bite or two of something indulgent. Then, eat it mindfully (page 31), savoring every sensation to enjoy it to the fullest. Knowing that something you crave isn't forbidden will decrease the power it has over you.

Get back on track

Nobody's perfect. Sometimes you'll be at a party where the food and fun are just too amazing to resist; or you'll oversleep instead of doing the morning workout you committed to; or you didn't have time to cook a healthful meal and had to make a quick stop at the nearest fast-food joint.

These are moments to remember one of the most important truths of successful weight management: *Lapses are not the end of the world.* You can get right back on track with small, simple compensations. If you ate too much last night or missed your workout yesterday, today is the perfect chance for you to start anew.

Power through the Last Few Pounds

It's a weight-management wish you've probably heard, or said to yourself, many times: "I really want to lose those last five (or ten) pounds, but they just won't seem to go away." There are several logical reasons why people managing their weight reach such a plateau. And there are some easy strategies you can follow that may help you get back on track to reaching your goal.

ADJUST YOUR CALORIE INTAKE A lighter body needs fewer calories to maintain its weight. For example, after a weight loss of 25 pounds, a person could need on average 200 calories less per day. People who don't decrease the amount of calories they eat may find that weight loss slows. To counteract this phenomenon, always be sure to keep a detailed record of what you eat every day using a food journal (pages 52–53 and the sample journal pages you'll find on pages 232–233), along with the nutritional information you'll find accompanying the recipes in this book as well as on food packaging and in calorie tables. Then, every time you lose five or ten pounds, make adjustments to your daily total calorie goal.

DOUBLE-CHECK PORTION SIZES Sometimes, after people have some success dropping pounds, they may gradually become less diligent about measuring portion sizes. Are you still checking your portion sizes carefully, or have you become more casual with measuring? Without even noticing, you could be eating more than you need, even of the healthful foods. Get out those measuring cups and scales and keep them on your kitchen counter. Review the goals in MyPyramid and the common portion size comparisons (pages 24–25; page 31) so they'll stay fresh in your mind when you're eating out.

BEWARE OF EXTRA CALORIES It's possible that you're consuming extra calories by not measuring while you cook, by idly nibbling or dipping, or having "just one more" sugary or alcoholic drink. For example, using just one extra tablespoon of olive oil when sautéing or drizzled onto your bread plate adds 120 calories; drinking just one sugary soda or extra glass of wine is around 100–150 calories. You also may be adding calories by absentmindedly reaching into office snack bowls, or finishing pizza crusts your child leaves on the plate. The solution to this mindless eating is simple: Make the effort to become more aware of these kinds of behaviors, training yourself to jot down in your food journal every single thing you eat or drink.

WRITE DOWN EVERYTHING Resume the practice of writing down everything you eat. If you don't have your journal pages with you, record what you consume on your computer or smartphone. Be sure to look over your journal or notes at the end of every day so that you are more aware of what you've been eating and can recognize any changes you may need to make.

REDEDICATE YOURSELF TO EXERCISE Some people let weight-management success be an excuse to ease up on workouts. Others fall into routines that become boring, or that they practice so efficiently that their bodies no longer burn as many calories as they used to. Your weight-loss plateau may be partly caused by the fact that you're simply no longer getting as much exercise as you need—or getting as much benefit as you used to out of the exercise you've been doing. You can easily address this situation, too. First, review the basic principles of exercise for weight management (pages 36–41). Then, with the help of a fitness trainer or other expert, and the advice and approval of your doctor, increase your exercise intensity and frequency, aiming for 60 minutes most days.

RECONSIDER YOUR GOAL The last explanation is the simplest of all: *You may not need to lose those final pounds.* You may have already reached a weight that's healthy for you! To find out, calculate your Body Mass Index (page 11) to see if your weight now falls within the range of healthy. Then, ask yourself how well and energetic you feel instead of what you think the scale should say.

Challenge yourself

If you want to give your weight-management efforts a fresh start, always remember that you can enlist the help of **The Special K Challenge**™ (pages 13–19) up to three times per year. Especially for resolutions, swimsuit season and to drop a jeans size, women everywhere know that **Special K**® foods can be the weight-management partner that gets them back on track nutritiously, deliciously and with satisfaction.*

*Consult your physician before starting any diet or exercise program. Average weight loss when replacing meals with two cereal meals is 4.8 pounds. Average waist circumference reduction when replacing meals with two cereal meals is 1.3 inches. Weight loss may vary.

Keep a Weight-Management Journal

Research has shown that keeping track daily of everything you eat and drink as well as of what exercise you do and what progress you've achieved can be an effective way to stay on track with your weight-management plan. Jotting down the details of your journey can help you stay motivated. It can also keep you constantly more aware of your goals and what you can do to make progress toward them most effectively. On a more basic level, the simple act of writing things down can help you get a greater feeling of being in control. And that, in turn, may lead to positive, long-lasting results.

A study published in the August 2008 issue of the American Journal of Preventive Medicine *followed the weight-loss journeys of 1,685 people. All of them participated in weekly programs that focused on healthful eating and exercise. Some were also required to keep daily records of what they ate and how much they exercised. After six months, those who kept journals lost twice as much weight as those who didn't.*

Pre-printed, photocopy-ready, fill-in-the-blanks journal pages like those in this book (pages 232–233) can help many people stay more organized and dedicated to writing things down on their weight-management journey. (See the opposite page for basic guidelines for getting the most out of those pages.)

If you prefer, feel free to find another approach that works for you. Maybe you'll choose a bound blank journal or diary with a beautiful cover, or an old-fashioned school binder or a file on your computer. Or maybe you'd rather jot down the details on sticky notes or a small notebook you keep with you wherever you go. Others might prefer using the note-taking feature or an application on a smartphone; some applications can calculate calories in a meal, suggest healthful seasonal ingredients and provide a journaling platform in an interactive all-in-one format.

Whatever method you choose, you'll improve your odds of reaching and maintaining your ideal weight by writing things down. Reading your journal from time to time can help you track your progress, identify areas that need more attention and help you recognize—and celebrate—your victories.

TIPS ON JOURNALING

It's easy to create your own weight-management journal. Just make multiple photocopies of the journal pages you'll find on pages 232–233. Punch holes in them if you like, and then keep them in a notebook or a folder. Follow these simple tips to help you get the most out of the journal pages—or from any other journaling system you choose to use.

Log what you eat and drink Jot down everything—meals, snacks and beverages. Don't forget to record any casual nibbles you might take throughout the day. Include portion sizes (pages 24–25, 31) and, if counting them helps, calories. There's a space to fill in a daily calorie goal. Ask your doctor, a registered dietitian or other weight-management expert, or consult an online resource, for specific goals for your height, build and activity level.

Record how much you exercise Write down your physical activity, whether it's a brisk walk, taking the stairs, housecleaning, going to the gym, or exercising outdoors or in front of your TV (pages 36–41). Every time you complete ten minutes or more of physical activity, write it down.

Indicate your weight Weigh yourself regularly—first thing in the morning before you eat—and write it down so you can chart your progress or nip setbacks in the bud. Don't feel you have to weigh yourself every day, especially if natural day-to-day fluctuations discourage you.

Note your measurements Even when the scale doesn't show it, your measurements can help you chart your progress and feel victorious. Check regularly with a tape measure and note those measurements.

Express how you're feeling It can help to jot down anything else you think is relevant. It could be foods you found hard to resist, or stressful situations that made you want to eat. Or, you may want to celebrate triumphs of self-control, or compliments you received, wonderful dreams you've had or activities that made you feel energetic, healthy and happy. Treat your journal pages as a personal diary.

Share your successes Share your journal pages with loved ones or friends who are supporting you—or joining you—on your weight-management journey. A fresh pair of eyes may notice things you might want to do differently for even greater results. And a caring supporter will comfort you through any minor setbacks—and cheer you through your victories.

Cook for Weight Management

When you plan meals, shop for them, and prepare them for yourself, you literally take your weight management into your own hands. Success comes through choosing nutritious, healthful ingredients and then cooking them in ways that make the most of their natural flavors and textures while minimizing fat and salt.

Just as keeping a food journal plays an important role in managing your weight (pages 52–53), so too does planning healthful meals. Schedule one or two weeks' worth of menus—meal by meal and snack by snack—and you'll find it easier to stay on track every day. Meal planning doesn't mean denying yourself treats—just schedule in the possibility for enjoying them now and then, making adjustments to the rest of your day's or week's plans.

To help you with meal planning, refer to MyPyramid (pages 24–25) and the recipes in this book (pages 65–231). But if you're someone who usually takes a more casual approach to organization, you can still aim to have ingredients on hand for a week's or more meals without deciding ahead of time what you'll cook and eat on any given day. Planning ahead will still help you make sure that you have healthful, delicious ingredients available and ready to prepare. Whatever your personality, the following tips can help you plan healthful meals more successfully.

CREATE A MENU PLAN On the weekend, create a meal-planning template, day by day, for the next week or more, leaving spaces to fill in for each meal and snack. You can use a sheet of blank paper, preprinted calendar pages or a menu-planning template found online. For convenience, rely on healthful favorites that you repeat as often as you and your family like. Aim to enjoy a variety of ingredients from MyPyramid (pages 24–25) to keep your meals varied and meet your nutritional needs.

SHOP FOR SMART STAPLES By keeping some basics on hand, you'll be able to whip up last-minute meals when you don't have time to cook or don't feel like making what you've scheduled. Stock your freezer and pantry with items such as frozen vegetables and fruits, lean ground meat and poultry, low-sodium broth, pasta, rice, canned beans, canned water-packed tuna, canned tomatoes, canola and olive oils and cereals.

COOK AHEAD Cook large-batch recipes, such as soups, stews, casseroles and pasta sauces, on the weekend and freeze extra in individual meal-sized containers, ready for quick reheating midweek. Prepare small containers to pack for lunches, too.

DECIPHERING NUTRITION FACTS

The black-and-white Nutrition Facts panels on the sides of packaged foods, and the brief nutritional analyses included with the recipes in this book provide a wide range of information about nutrients. In general, here's the information you should focus on based on 2,000 calories per day. Ask your doctor for goals tailored specifically to your own height, weight, age and body type.

Serving size To ensure you don't serve yourself a larger portion than you need, pay attention to the serving size listed on packages or the number of servings for recipes. Each recipe in this book yields portions that are consistent in size with USDA guidelines.

Calories If you're counting them (page 29), keep track of the calories per serving in your food journal. Aim for no more in a day than the desired amount for your height and activity level.

Calories from fat Aim overall for no more than about one-third of daily calories from fat, balancing higher-fat recipes or ingredients with those that are lower in fat. To calculate the percentage of calories from fat, divide the number of fat calories listed by the total calories, and then move the decimal point two places to the right.

Total fat Aim for less than 65g of fat per day. Whenever possible, strive for foods that include monounsaturated fat or polyunsaturated fat, both of which, in moderation, have been found to help prevent heart disease.

Saturated fat Aim for no more than 20g of saturated fat per day. Excessive intake of saturated fat has been linked to an increased risk of cardiovascular disease and certain cancers.

Trans fat Limit as much as possible your intake of trans fats found in processed foods containing hydrogenated vegetable fats. They have been linked to an increased risk of heart disease.

Cholesterol Aim to consume less than 300mg per day of cholesterol, found in foods of animal origin and especially in organ meats, shellfish, and egg yolks.

Sodium Aim for less than 2,300mg per day (note that 1,500mg per day is considered adequate).

Carbohydrates Aim for a total of 300g of carbohydrates, including nutrient- and fiber-rich whole grains.

Dietary fiber Aim for at least 25g fiber.

Sugars Limit the sugars you eat and cook with, treating them as part of your "Discretionary Calories" on MyPyramid.

Proteins Aim for 10 to 15 percent of your daily calories from protein (50 to 75g).

Shop for Healthful Foods

Once you've planned your menus for a week or more (page 54), grocery shopping can be a breeze. You may only need to shop every other week, with occasional stops for perishable items. From your menu plans, you'll easily be able to create a shopping list (page 59), organizing it by supermarket departments. List in hand, you're ready to go shopping. Whenever you shop, go only after you've eaten a meal.

Studies show that hungry shoppers tend to buy more food and make less healthful choices than shoppers who are satiated. Hungry shoppers also tend to give into temptation when standing in the checkout line surrounded by the candy commonly displayed near the cash register.

Shop the perimeter of the store for most of the ingredients you'll need to cook for your third meal when you're on **The Special K Challenge™,** or for the key ingredients in most of your main dishes and side dishes when you're preparing three meals a day. That's where you'll find fresh vegetables and fruits; dairy products; and seafood, poultry and meats. Then, head strategically to other aisles for the staples you need: **Special K®** cereals, protein bars and snacks; whole grains and dried beans; canned goods including low-sodium broths, canned tomatoes and water-packed tuna or salmon; and healthy frozen foods such as fruits and vegetables and unprocessed seafood and poultry. With your menu plan and shopping list filled out, and comfortably satisfied with healthful food, here are some more strategies to help you shop smartly.

GRAINS MyPyramid recommends three servings of whole grains daily, not just for their fiber content but also for essential vitamins, minerals and other nutrients. Look for cereals (such as **Special K** cereals), breads and crackers that feature whole grains. Choose staple grains such as pearl barley, bulgur wheat, quinoa and brown rice to serve as healthful side dishes.

VEGETABLES AND FRUIT Whether you're in the supermarket produce section or at the farmers' market, look not only for your own year-round favorites, but also for vegetables and fruits at their seasonal best, some of which you might not have tried before. Grab some fresh herbs, too, to add extra color and flavor to your meals. Consider, too, stopping by the freezer section. Having a few bags of frozen produce on hand— pretrimmed, precut and ready to cook—will help ensure you never go without fruits and vegetables. In addition, some frozen products may even be more nutrient-rich than fresh options, because they're frozen soon after picking at their peak.

DAIRY Choose fat-free (skim) or low-fat (1%) milk and yogurt. With yogurt, buying plain varieties and adding your own fresh fruit or other flavorings enables you to control how much sugar you add while also saving some money. In general, choose cheeses labeled "low-fat" (3g or less of fat per serving), "reduced-fat" (25 percent less fat than its full-fat version) or "fat-free" (less than 0.5g fat per serving). If you're watching your sodium intake, look for cheeses labeled "reduced-sodium." If your cholesterol level isn't a concern, you may opt for regular-fat cheeses, but eat them in moderation. Note, too, that many full-fat cheeses are also fuller in flavor than their low-fat counterparts, making a small portion, savored slowly, more satisfying than a larger portion of low-fat or fat-free cheese.

EGGS Whether organic, free-range, brown-shelled, or white, the nutrients in hens' eggs are virtually identical. Eggs are an excellent, inexpensive source of protein, and provide choline, a nutrient essential for the central nervous system and vitamin D. True, egg yolks are high in cholesterol, with one large yolk containing about 215mg. But, depending on what your doctor advises and what else you eat in a given day, that still means you could eat one egg a day and stay below the recommended limit of 300mg of cholesterol daily. Cooking eggs is among the quickest, easiest ways to get a meal on the table, but you also have the option in many recipes of using fat-free egg whites alone or substituting commercial fat- and cholesterol-free pasteurized egg products that look and taste like beaten whole eggs.

SEAFOOD Variety is the best approach to buying and eating seafood. This way, you'll consume fish of varying levels of heart-healthy omega-3 fatty acids (highest in higher-fat, cold-water fish like albacore tuna, Atlantic herring, lake trout, mackerel, salmon, sardines and swordfish) without overdependence on any one. When buying fresh fish, ask what choices are freshest the day you shop, and ask for substitutions if what you're looking for is unavailable. Look online, too, for suggestions for sustainable, environmentally responsible seafood choices. Many economical options can also be found in the freezer section. Still more good choices include canned salmon, sardines and water-packed albacore tuna.

POULTRY Poultry is high in protein and generally low in fat. Boneless, skinless chicken breasts have become the go-to meat for those on a weight-management plan, but their mild flavor can seem a little lackluster to eaters who enjoy bold flavors. Dark-meat chicken thighs are a flavorful substitute, with their deeper flavor and fuller texture. Remove poultry skin, which has a lot of excess fat, before or after cooking. Ground poultry can be deceiving; check the fat percentage for the lowest available. Economical whole chickens and turkeys can be roasted and the meat frozen for countless meal-planning options. Use or freeze all raw poultry promptly after purchase to avoid it becoming a food safety concern.

MEAT Red meat can be higher in calories and fat than many seafood choices or skinless white-meat poultry, but sometimes, a meal of red meat satisfies cravings like nothing else. It also provides lots of protein, B vitamins, iron and zinc. Choose leaner beef cuts from the round or loin sections, and lamb or pork from the loin or leg. Beef labeled "Select" grade will be leaner than "Choice" or top "Prime" cuts, which are marbled with more fat. Plan on about four ounces of uncooked, boneless meat per person, which will yield a three-ounce cooked serving size.

BEANS AND LENTILS These are satisfying nutritional powerhouses, low in fat and packed with protein, fiber and complex carbohydrates. Their mild, earthy flavors invite a wide variety of creative seasonings. Whenever time allows, start with dried beans, which are not only lower in sodium than most canned products, but also cost a fraction of the price of canned per serving.

Quick-soaking beans

Don't have enough time to soak dried beans overnight—or didn't plan ahead? Try this convenient quick-soak method: Rinse the dried beans in a colander under cold running water. Place them in a large pot with six cups cold water for every pound of beans. Bring to a full rolling boil over high heat and continue boiling for two minutes. Remove from the heat, cover, and let stand at room temperature for one hour. Drain the beans well, cover with fresh, cold water, and simmer until tender, about one hour.

SHOPPING LIST

Preparing a shopping list before you head for the market will help you make sure that you buy only the healthful foods you need, avoiding impulse purchases. Use this form as a starting point, comparing the list to the recipes you plan to cook and to the contents of your pantry and refrigerator.

Grains

- ☐ **Special K®** cereals
- ☐ Brown rice
- ☐ Couscous, quick cooking
- ☐ Pasta, whole wheat
- ☐ Tortillas (whole wheat, spinach or corn)
- ☐ _____
- ☐ _____

Vegetables

- ☐ Beans
- ☐ Broccoli
- ☐ Bell peppers
- ☐ Bok Choy
- ☐ Carrots
- ☐ Herbs
- ☐ Lettuce
- ☐ Mushrooms
- ☐ Onions
- ☐ Potatoes
- ☐ Spinach
- ☐ Squashes, winter
- ☐ Sweet potatoes
- ☐ Zucchini
- ☐ _____
- ☐ _____

Fruit

- ☐ Apples
- ☐ Bananas
- ☐ Berries
- ☐ Melons
- ☐ Oranges
- ☐ Peaches
- ☐ Pears
- ☐ _____
- ☐ _____

Eggs & dairy

- ☐ Eggs
- ☐ Fat-free egg product
- ☐ Low-fat cheese
- ☐ Nonfat or low-fat milk
- ☐ Nonfat plain yogurt
- ☐ _____
- ☐ _____

Seafood, poultry & meat

- ☐ Beef, extra-lean, ground
- ☐ Beef sirloin
- ☐ Chicken breasts, boneless, skinless
- ☐ Fish, mild, white
- ☐ Pork tenderloin
- ☐ Salmon
- ☐ Shrimp
- ☐ Tuna, fresh
- ☐ Turkey breast cutlets
- ☐ Turkey, ground
- ☐ _____
- ☐ _____

Canned goods

- ☐ Broth, reduced sodium
- ☐ Tomatoes
- ☐ Tuna, water-packed
- ☐ _____
- ☐ _____

Staples & snacks

- ☐ Beans, dried
- ☐ Dressings, fat-free or reduced-fat
- ☐ Soy sauce, reduced-sodium
- ☐ **Special K** snacks and crackers
- ☐ **Special K** protein bars
- ☐ **Special K** protein shakes
- ☐ _____
- ☐ _____

Basics of Healthy Cooking

Cooking for yourself and your loved ones makes it easy for you to enjoy delicious meals that are not only packed with nutrients but also low in calories, fat and sodium. But there's another benefit as well: When you cook good food, you start enjoying it long before you sit down to eat. From shopping for beautiful, fresh vegetables and fruit, to preparing the ingredients with care, to experiencing the wonderful aromas and even hearing the sounds of your food as it cooks, every step provides an opportunity for enjoyment. What better, more pleasurable way could there be to manage your weight? And by cooking your own meals, you can really improve your chances of weight-management success.

> *According to a survey published by the Consumer Reports National Research Center in 2009, the more days per week survey respondents said they ate restaurant or takeout dinners, the greater their weight.*

As long as you've planned your meals smartly and have on hand the ingredients you need (pages 54–59), cooking at home can also be quick and easy. The recipes on the pages that follow have been developed specifically to yield great results even for inexperienced home cooks, using widely available ingredients, simple preparation techniques and straightforward, healthy cooking methods.

BAKING With hardly any work on your part, the dry heat of your oven can perform delicious feats, such as turning crumb-coated chicken cutlets (page 133) as crisp on the outside and juicy within as if they'd been deep-fried in oil. Baking can also turn fresh fruit tender, soft and sweet for desserts like Baked Apples with Almond-Apricot Filling (page 214). Whatever the recipe, be sure to allow 10 to 15 minutes for the oven to preheat. Line baking pans with aluminum foil or parchment paper for easy cleanup. If you need a greased pan, coat it lightly with nonstick cooking spray.

BRAISING This slow, moist cooking method involves cooking larger pieces of food to tenderness in a relatively small amount of gently simmering liquid in a tightly covered vessel. Done on the stove top or in the oven, braising is great for less-tender cuts of meat or poultry, such as in Braised Turkey Thighs with Winter Root Vegetables (page 155).

BROILING Cooking fairly small, thin, tender pieces of food with very intense, dry heat from above cooks them quickly, producing a richly browned, flavorful surface and juicy interior. Preheat the broiler for 10 to 15 minutes before you start cooking, and keep a regular watch to avoid burning. Broiling can take the place of an outdoor grill in the event of inclement weather in such recipes as Blackened Salmon-and-Vegetable Kabobs (page 98).

GRILLING You can cook an entire meal on the grill while keeping cleanup to a minimum. And grilling doesn't need to be confined to the warmer months anymore. You can enjoy healthful, satisfying recipes like Grilled Chicken Salad (page 143) year round, thanks to convenient indoor grills, ridged stove top grill pans, and counter top hinged electric "contact" grills (which, applying heat from both sides at once, cook grilled recipes in half the time). Whatever grill you use, follow the manufacturer's instructions carefully for best results.

POACHING No added fat is needed for this technique, in which an already tender ingredient, such as the star of Apple-Cherry Poached Chicken (page 132), is quickly cooked when partially or completely submerged in gently simmering liquid. Being such a gentle cooking method, poaching is also ideal for delicate foods that easily fall apart or dry out, such as flaky white fish.

ROASTING Both large cuts of meat or poultry and big pieces of vegetables cook beautifully in the dry heat of an oven set to moderate heat, turning tender and juicy within while developing a richly browned surface. You'll be amazed by how, by caramelizing their natural sugars, roasting can transform the flavors of vegetables you might consider commonplace. Roasted Cauliflower and Tomatoes (page 196) is a perfect example.

SAUTÉING Similar to stir-frying, this classic technique quickly sears small or thin pieces of food to doneness in a skillet or sauté pan over high heat, using just a little oil or nonstick cooking spray. Working in combination with seasonings, the high heat gives dishes like Sautéed Shrimp Tacos (page 116) vivid flavor, and the juices that caramelize on the bottom of the pan can be deglazed to create a delicious pan sauce, as in Sautéed Veal with Balsamic Sauce (page 168).

STEAMING Naturally tender food cooks wonderfully, without added fat, when suspended in a steamer basket or wire steamer and surrounded by steam, or when sealed inside parchment paper or foil and baked in the oven. Use steaming to cook vegetables until just slightly crisp or delicate fish fillets, like Mustard-Topped Halibut in Parchment (page 114), to perfect doneness.

STEWING Closely related to braising, stewing employs the same slow, moist cooking technique to small pieces of food. It does wonders to lean, less-tender cuts of meat and poultry, such as the top round in Beef Stew with Mushrooms (page 163) or the stew meat in Pork Posole (page 173).

STIR-FRYING This method of quickly cooking food over high heat while stirring constantly maintains the crispness of fresh vegetables and the tenderness of meat in dishes like Sichuan Orange Beef-and-Broccoli Stir-Fry (page 158). Stir-frying is a speedy and healthful way to get dinner on the table, but it does require some diligent preparation and hands-on cooking. Start with tender cuts of meat or poultry, or pieces of firm seafood like shrimp or scallops, and quick-cooking vegetables cut into uniform bite-sized pieces for even cooking. Preheat a wok or large skillet over medium-high to high heat, and then add just a little oil or nonstick spray. Start adding those ingredients that take longest to cook and keep them moving continuously around the pan as you stir with a long-handled spatula or spoon.

Tools for healthy cooking

You don't need specialized cooking equipment to make healthful meals.

Baking and roasting Large baking sheets, roasting pan or baking dish

Braising and stewing Dutch oven, large saucepan or soup pot with a cover

Broiling Two-part broiler pan or rimmed baking sheet

Grilling Outdoor charcoal or gas grill or specialized indoor grill

Poaching Large saucepan or Dutch oven

Sautéing and stir-frying Large frying pan or wok

Steaming Saucepan with steamer insert or strainer

KITCHEN SAFETY TIPS

Along with always using common sense, take care when preparing meals to ensure that your food is wholesome. The following kitchen tips will help you keep your food delicious and healthful when you cook at home.

Handle with care Be especially cautious when handling knives and other sharp tools. When you handle hot cookware, use dry pot holders or dry oven mitts. Keep long sleeves rolled up and long hair safely tied back. Let hot cookware cool before putting it into the sink. Clean up spills right away.

Keep ingredients separate Keep raw, cooked and ready-to-eat foods separate from each other to avoid the possibility of cross-contamination from any harmful bacteria. Never place cooked food on a plate that previously held raw meat, poultry, or seafood.

Keep hands and surfaces clean Before and after you handle food, wash your hands thoroughly with lots of warm, soapy water and then rinse well. Do the same for any surfaces, dishes or implements that come into contact with food.

Rinse fresh foods before preparing Wash all fruits and vegetables with cold water, while scrubbing sturdy items with a soft-bristled vegetable brush. There's no need for you to rinse meat or poultry; doing so can actually spread any bacteria, which will be destroyed by heat when you cook the food to recommended safe temperatures (see right).

Store cooked foods sensibly Transfer hot foods you plan to store to a refrigerator container and then put straight into the refrigerator; there's no need to cool them first. Refrigerate prepared foods or leftover take-out within two hours or sooner.

Use a food thermometer When you cook large pieces of meat or poultry, use an instant-read thermometer to check for doneness. Near the end of cooking time, insert the tip into the thickest part of the food (not touching any bone or fat or gristle). If necessary, keep checking regularly until the food reaches the recommended minimum safe internal temperature as shown below. As with other kitchen tools, wash the thermometer with hot, soapy water after each use.

USDA safe cooking temperatures:
- Steaks/roasts/chops 145°F
- Seafood 145°F
- Pork 160°F
- Ground meats 160°F
- Egg dishes 160°F
- Chicken breasts 165°F
- Whole poultry 165°F

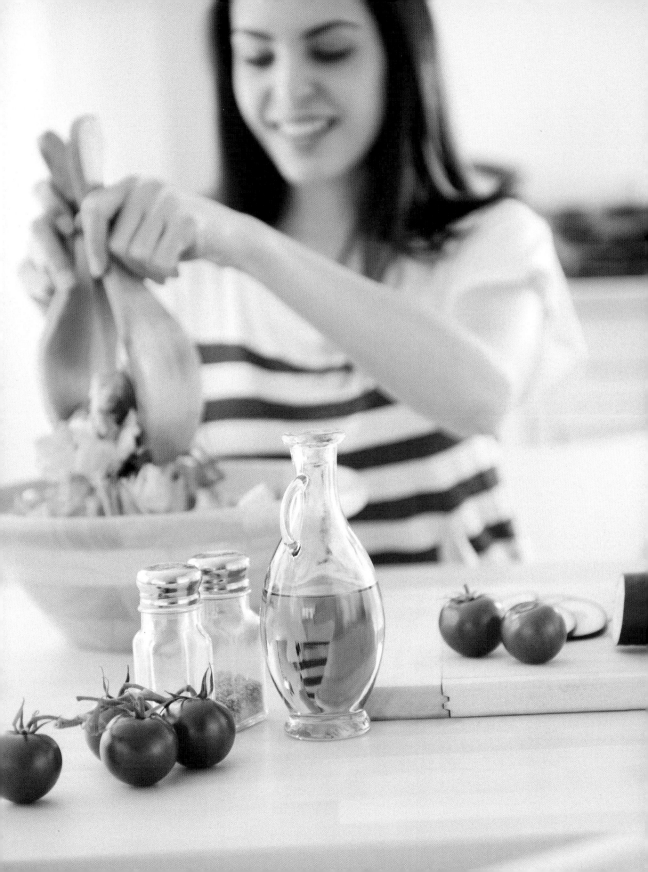

Cook your way to victory

One of the questions fans of **The Special K Challenge**™ ask most frequently is, "What should I cook for my third meal?" That question is easy to answer: Eat a normal, healthful meal featuring delicious food like the recipes on the following pages—the same kinds of nutrient-packed, satisfying fare that you normally enjoy. Along with **Special K**® foods and sensible snacks, you can continue toward your weight-management goal well beyond **The Special K Challenge.** Here's wishing you happy—and healthful—eating!

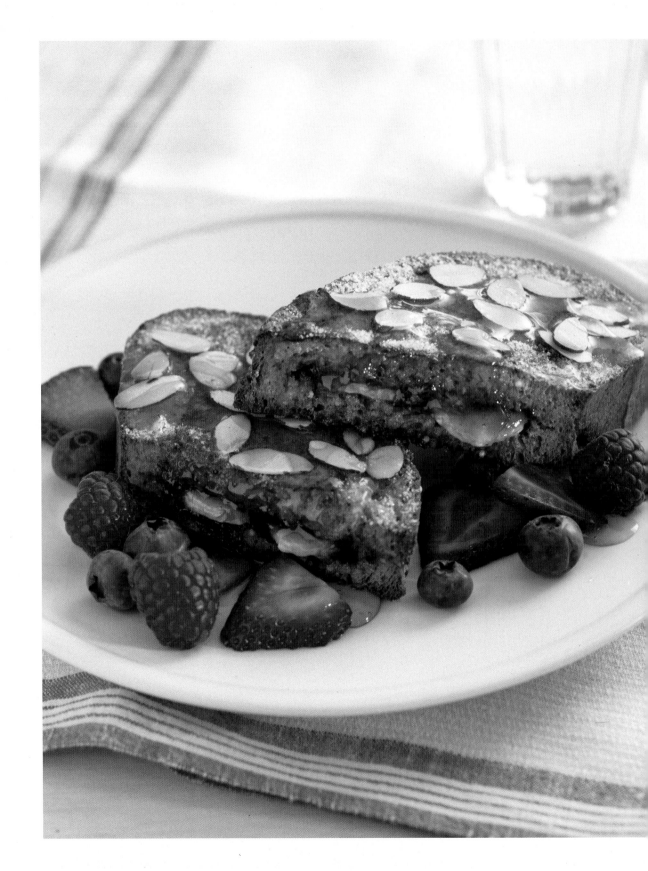

Breakfast and Brunch

Spinach-Feta Frittata

1½ cups refrigerated fat-free egg product

¼ cup nonfat milk

1 teaspoon dried dill

¼ teaspoon salt

¼ teaspoon pepper

½ cup finely chopped onions

1 clove garlic, minced

2 teaspoons vegetable oil

3 cups fresh baby spinach

¼ cup crumbled reduced-fat feta cheese

Although this Italian omelet, loaded with fresh spinach and topped with feta cheese, is wonderful for weekend mornings, it also makes a great casual weeknight supper.

1 Preheat broiler.

2 In medium mixing bowl whisk together egg product, milk, dill, salt and pepper. Set aside.

3 In large skillet cook onions and garlic in oil over medium heat until tender, stirring occasionally. Add spinach. Cook, stirring frequently, for 1 to 2 minutes or until wilted.

4 Pour egg mixture over spinach in skillet. Cook over medium heat. As mixture begins to set, run spatula around edges, allowing uncooked portions to flow underneath. Continue until egg mixture is almost set.

5 Sprinkle with feta cheese. Broil 4 to 5 inches from heat for 2 to 3 minutes or until frittata is lightly browned and completely set. To serve, cut into wedges and serve immediately or lukewarm.

NUTRITION FACTS PER SERVING Calories: 100; Calories from Fat: 30; **Total Fat:** 3g; **Saturated Fat:** 0.5g; **Trans Fat:** 0g; **Cholesterol:** 5mg; **Sodium:** 460mg; **Total Carbohydrate:** 7g; **Dietary Fiber:** 1g; **Sugars:** 3g; **Protein:** 12g

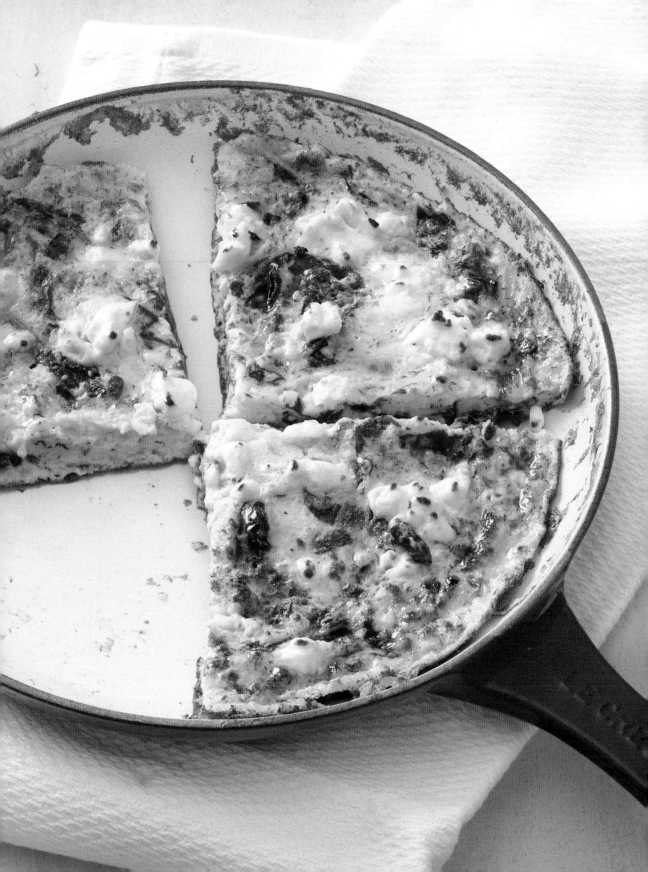

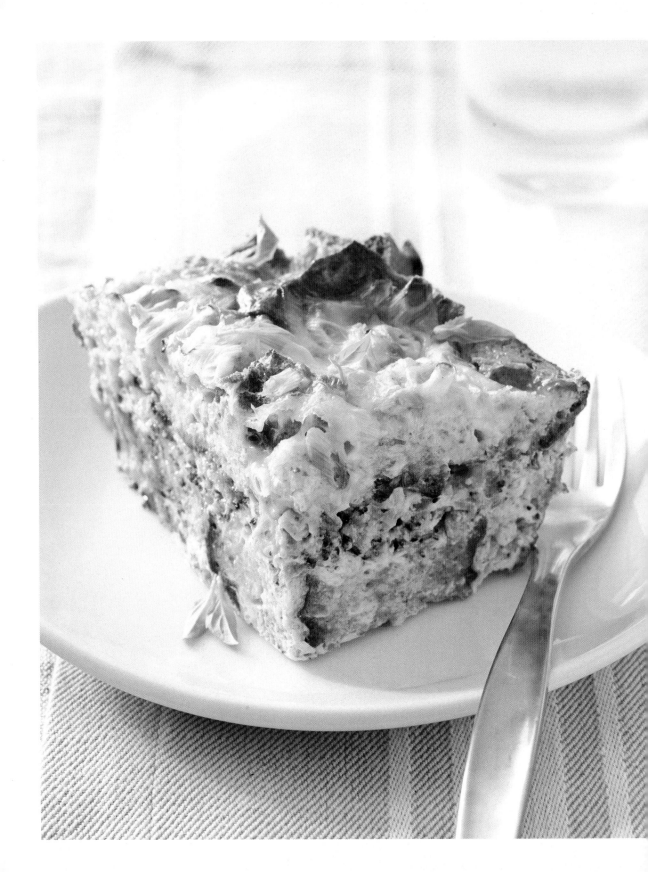

Provolone-Broccoli Strata

1½ cups finely chopped
fresh broccoli

2 tablespoons water

Butter-flavored
cooking spray

5 cups multigrain
or whole-wheat
baguette cubes

1 cup shredded aged
provolone cheese

½ cup finely chopped
Canadian-style bacon
(about 2 ounces)

1 tablespoon chopped
fresh basil or 1 teaspoon
dried basil leaves

½ cup sliced
green onions

2 cups refrigerated
fat-free egg product

1 cup fat-free
half-and-half

½ teaspoon dry mustard

¼ teaspoon pepper

⅛ teaspoon salt

Assemble this satisfying Italian-style savory bread pudding before you go to bed; the next day, it will be ready to pop in the oven to become the star of your weekend brunch.

1 In 1-quart microwave-safe casserole combine broccoli and water. Micro-cook, covered, at high for 2 minutes. Drain well.

2 In 8 x 8 x 2-inch baking dish coated with cooking spray, layer half of the bread. Sprinkle with broccoli. Top with half of the cheese, and all of the bacon and basil. Layer remaining bread, remaining cheese and onions on top.

3 In medium bowl whisk together egg product, half-and-half, mustard, pepper and salt. Slowly pour over mixture in baking dish. Lightly press bread down into egg mixture. Cover with plastic wrap and refrigerate for 4 to 24 hours.

4 Preheat oven to 350°F. Bake, uncovered, for 45 to 55 minutes or until knife inserted near center comes out clean. Let stand for 5 minutes. To serve, cut into squares.

NUTRITION FACTS PER SERVING **Calories:** 240; **Calories from Fat:** 60; **Total Fat:** 6g; **Saturated Fat:** 3.5g; **Trans Fat:** 0g; **Cholesterol:** 20mg; **Sodium:** 740mg; **Total Carbohydrate:** 24g; **Dietary Fiber:** 2g; **Sugars:** 6g; **Protein:** 20g

Strawberry AND Cheese Muffins

SERVES 12

¼ cup fat-free
cream cheese

2 tablespoons seedless
strawberry jam

1½ cups all-purpose flour

1 tablespoon
baking powder

¼ teaspoon salt

½ teaspoon cinnamon

2 cups **Kellogg's®**
Special K® Red
Berries cereal

½ cup sugar

1 cup nonfat plain
yogurt

2 egg whites

2 tablespoons
vegetable oil

Butter-flavored
cooking spray

¼ cup sliced almonds
(optional)

Almost like cheesecake for breakfast, these colorful treats are packed with satisfying flavor and texture. They're surprisingly low in fat and very easy to make.

1 Preheat oven to 400°F.

2 In small mixing bowl combine cream cheese and strawberry jam until thoroughly combined. Set aside.

3 In another bowl stir together flour, baking powder, salt and cinnamon. Set aside.

4 In large mixing bowl, combine **Special K** Red Berries cereal, sugar, yogurt, egg whites and oil. Beat until thoroughly combined. Add flour mixture, stirring only until combined.

5 Coat twelve 2½-inch muffin-pan cups with cooking spray. Spoon batter evenly among cups. With spoon, make indention in center of batter in each muffin-pan cup. Place a slightly rounded teaspoon of cream cheese mixture into each. Sprinkle with almonds if desired.

6 Bake in preheated oven about 20 minutes or until golden brown. Serve warm.

NUTRITION FACTS PER SERVING Calories: 150; **Calories from Fat:** 20; **Total Fat:** 0.25g; **Saturated Fat:** 0g; **Trans Fat:** 0g; **Cholesterol:** 0mg; **Sodium:** 250mg; **Total Carbohydrate:** 29g; **Dietary Fiber:** 1g; **Sugars:** 14g; **Protein:** 4g

Kellogg's® Special K® Bran Muffins

1¼ cups all-purpose flour

1 tablespoon baking powder

¼ teaspoon salt (optional)

1 cup **Kellogg's® Special K®** cereal

1½ cups **Kellogg's® All-Bran® Original** or **All-Bran® Bran Buds®** cereal

¼ cup firmly packed brown sugar

1⅓ cups nonfat milk

2 egg whites

3 tablespoons vegetable oil

Butter-flavored cooking spray

Special K cereal adds extra flavor and texture to a this low-fat version of a classic recipe. If you like, add ½ to ¾ cup of seedless raisins or chopped dried fruit to the batter.

1 Preheat oven to 400°F.

2 In mixing bowl, stir together flour, baking powder and salt. In large bowl, combine **Special K** and **All-Bran** cereals, brown sugar and milk. Let stand about 2 minutes or until cereal softens. Add egg whites and oil. Beat well. Add flour mixture, stirring only until combined.

3 Coat twelve 2½-inch muffin-pan cups with cooking spray. Spoon batter evenly among cups.

4 Bake in preheated oven about 20 minutes or until lightly browned. Serve warm.

Here's to your health

Foods with fiber can help keep the digestive tract healthy. With an appropriate diet, they also support heart health and may help manage blood glucose levels. Some breakfast cereals like the bran cereal in this recipe help provide fiber. Other sources include: whole-grain products like brown rice and whole-wheat bread or spaghetti; fruits including skin-on pears and apples, strawberries, blackberries, bananas and kiwi; lentils and beans; vegetables like Brussels sprouts, carrots and broccoli; and nuts and seeds including almonds, peanuts and sunflower seeds. Check Nutrition Facts panels for fiber content.

NUTRITION FACTS PER SERVING Calories: 130; **Calories from Fat:** 35; **Total Fat:** 4g; **Saturated Fat:** 0g; **Trans Fat:** 0g; **Cholesterol:** 0mg; **Sodium:** 220mg; **Total Carbohydrate:** 23g; **Dietary Fiber:** 3g; **Sugars:** 9g; **Protein:** 4g

Banana-Stuffed Multigrain French Toast

Four 1-inch-thick slices honey wheat bread

2 tablespoons apricot or strawberry spreadable fruit

1 small banana, sliced

1 cup refrigerated fat-free egg product

½ cup nonfat milk

3 tablespoons sugar

1 teaspoon vanilla extract

Butter-flavored cooking spray

¼ teaspoon ground cinnamon

2 tablespoons sliced almonds

1 cup fresh raspberries, blueberries or sliced strawberries

½ cup maple syrup, warmed

Get a delicious jump on your daily servings of fresh fruit by combining bananas and berries with French toast made from fiber-rich multigrain bread and fat-free egg product.

1 Preheat oven to 450°F.

2 Diagonally cut each bread slice in half. With a small sharp knife carefully cut pocket in each piece from the diagonal edge. Spoon fruit spread inside of pockets. Arrange banana slices in pockets.

3 In shallow dish stir together egg product, milk, 2 tablespoons of the sugar and vanilla. Soak stuffed bread slices in egg mixture, generously coating both sides. Place slices on 15 x 10 x 1-inch baking pan lined with foil and coated with cooking spray. Bake in preheated oven for 10 minutes.

4 Meanwhile, stir together the remaining sugar and cinnamon.

5 With a spatula turn bread slices. Sprinkle with cinnamon mixture and almonds. Continue baking for 4 to 6 minutes more or until golden brown. Transfer to serving plates. Serve with berries and syrup.

NUTRITION FACTS PER SERVING Calories: 410; Calories from Fat: 40; Total Fat: 4.5g; Saturated Fat: 1g; Trans Fat: 0g; Cholesterol: 0mg; Sodium: 430mg; Total Carbohydrate: 83g; Dietary Fiber: 6g; Sugars: 49g; Protein: 13g

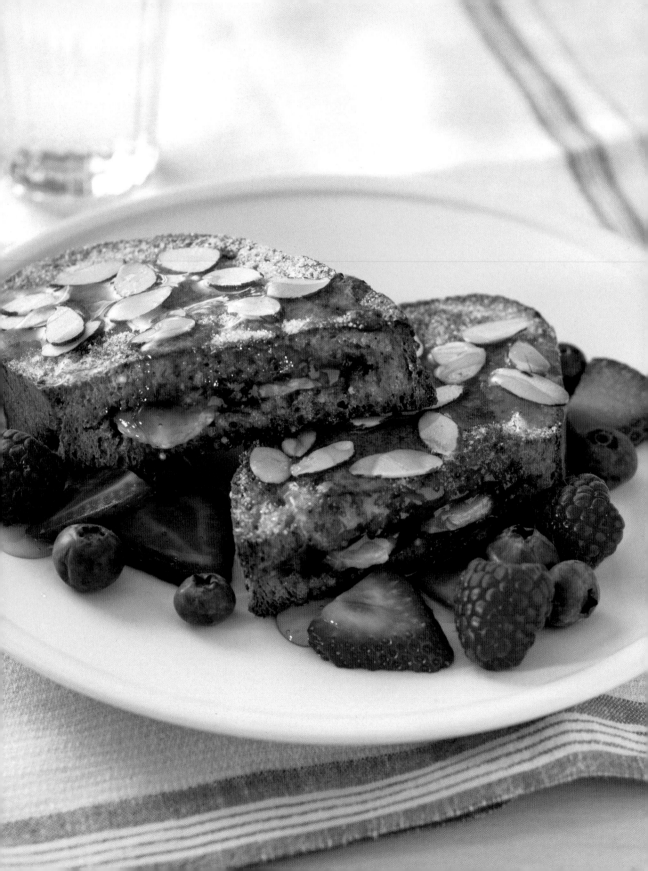

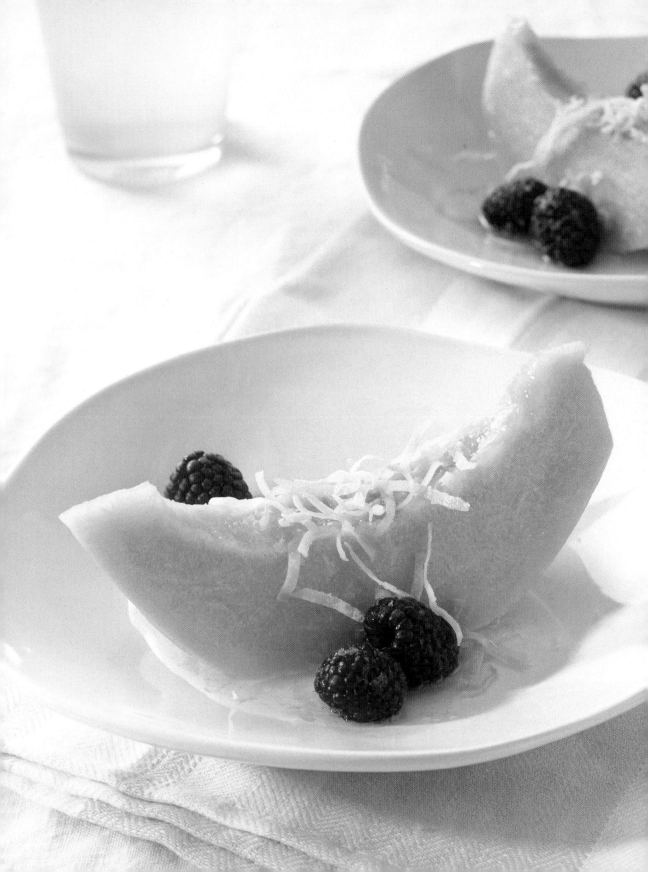

Gingered Cantaloupe
with Raspberries

SERVES 8

¾ cup water

½ cup sugar

4 teaspoons lemon juice

2 teaspoons grated
fresh ginger

1 teaspoon grated
lemon zest

1 small cantaloupe

1½ cups fresh raspberries

¼ cup shredded toasted
coconut (optional)

Hints of grated fresh ginger and lemon zest give cantaloupe and raspberries bright new appeal. If you like, you can cut the cantaloupe into cubes instead of serving it in wedges.

1 In saucepan stir together water, sugar, lemon juice and ginger. Bring to boiling. Reduce heat. Simmer, uncovered, for 3 minutes. Remove from heat. Stir in lemon zest. Cool to room temperature.

2 Halve cantaloupe. Scoop out seeds. Cut each half into 4 wedges. Trim rind from each wedge. Place each wedge in shallow soup plate or on serving plate. Sprinkle raspberries over cantaloupe. Pour sugar mixture over top. Sprinkle with coconut, if desired.

Here's to your health

Many orange-hued fresh fruits and vegetables are sources of beta-carotene, a nutrient your body converts into vitamin A. This powerful nutrient contributes to healthy skin, bone growth and vision. Good sources of beta-carotene include:

Fruits apricots, cantaloupes, mangoes, oranges, papayas and peaches

Vegetables carrots, dark leafy greens (such as kale, mustard greens and spinach), pumpkin and other winter squashes, and sweet potatoes

NUTRITION FACTS PER SERVING Calories: 80; Calories from Fat: 0; Total Fat: 0g; Saturated Fat: 0g; Trans Fat: 0g; Cholesterol: 0mg; **Sodium:** 10mg; **Total Carbohydrate:** 22g; **Dietary Fiber:** 1g; **Sugars:** 18g; **Protein:** 1g

Special K® Parfait

8 ounces low-fat vanilla-flavored yogurt

½ cup fresh fruit (sliced strawberries, sliced banana, blueberries or raspberries)

1 cup **Kellogg's®** **Special K®** cereal

Simple as can be, this beautiful and satisfying breakfast treat has long been a popular option to enjoy on **The Special K Challenge™.** Feel free to vary the fruit with the season.

1 In 2 tall glasses, layer spoonfuls of yogurt, fruit and **Special K** cereal until glasses are full.

2 Top with extra fruit and serve.

Make it a meal

Add these delicious side dishes to each serving to create a full meal (total additional calories: 350 per serving)

- 2 slices whole-wheat toast spread with 2 tablespoons peanut butter
- 8 ounces coffee or tea

NUTRITION FACTS PER SERVING **Calories:** 160; **Calories from Fat:** 15; **Total Fat:** 1.5g; **Saturated Fat:** 1g; **Trans Fat:** 0g; **Cholesterol:** 5mg; **Sodium:** 200mg; **Total Carbohydrate:** 30g; **Dietary Fiber:** 1g; **Sugars:** 19g; **Protein:** 9g

Peach Breakfast Smoothie

2 cups frozen, unsweetened peach slices

½ cup nonfat plain yogurt

½ cup nonfat milk

½ cup sugar

4 cups **Kellogg's®** **Special K®** Red Berries cereal

Need a healthful breakfast in a hurry? A smoothie is the perfect solution, especially when you pour it over a serving of one of your favorite **Special K** cereals.

1 Put peaches, yogurt, milk and sugar in food processor work bowl or blender container. Process until smooth, scraping down bowl or container sides occasionally.

2 Distribute **Special K** Red Berries cereal among 4 serving bowls. Pour smoothie mixture evenly over cereal. Serve immediately.

NUTRITION FACTS PER SERVING Calories: 200; Calories from Fat: 0; **Total Fat:** 0g; **Saturated Fat:** 0g; **Trans Fat:** 0g; **Cholesterol:** 0mg; **Sodium:** 240mg; **Total Carbohydrate:** 63g; **Dietary Fiber:** 4g; **Sugars:** 44g; **Protein:** 6g

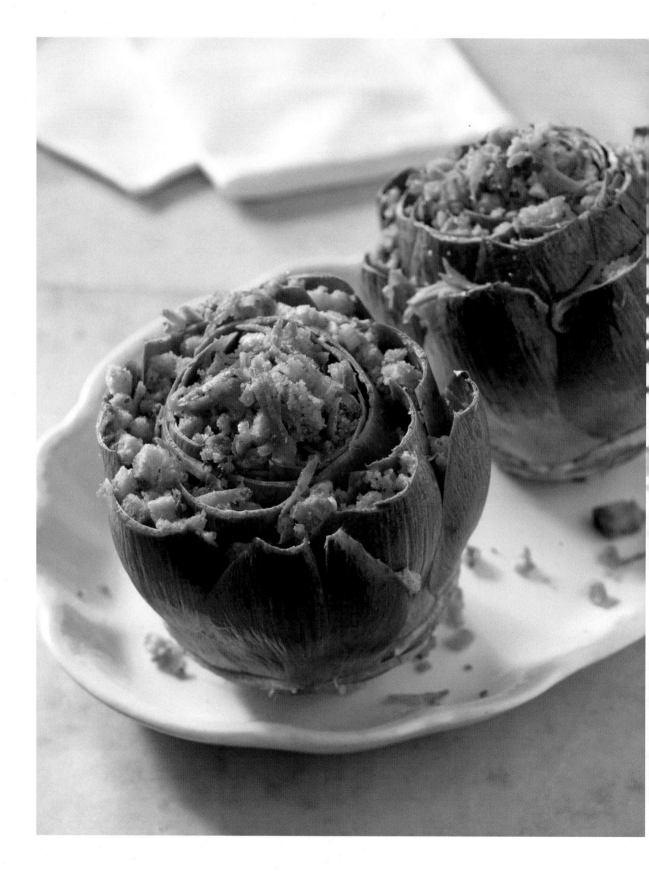

Appetizers and Soups

Tuscan Tomato-Bread Salad 82

Asparagus Salad with Citrus Dressing 85

Black Bean and Corn Dip with Oven-Baked Chips 86

Caesar Salad with Creamy Dressing 87

Cannellini Bean and Spinach Soup 88

Winter Minestrone 90

Chilled Cucumber-Mint Soup 91

Artichokes with Carrot-Cornbread Stuffing 93

Enlightened Guacamole 94

Lemon-Chive Ricotta Dip 95

Tuscan Tomato-Bread Salad

⅓ cup bottled fat-free
Italian salad dressing

2 tablespoons chopped
fresh basil

4 teaspoons red
wine vinegar

1 tablespoon grated
Parmesan cheese

¼ teaspoon coarsely
ground black pepper

4 cups multigrain
French baguette cubes
(about 1-inch cubes)

4 cups torn
romaine lettuce

2 cups coarsely
chopped tomatoes

1½ cups seeded and
coarsely chopped
cucumber

⅓ cup finely chopped
red onion

¼ cup pitted Kalamata
olives, chopped

For a great, easy salad dressing that tastes homemade, start with a store-bought fat-free dressing and customize it with your favorite tangy vinegar and fresh herbs.

1 Preheat oven to 325°F.

2 Meanwhile, for dressing, in small bowl whisk together Italian salad dressing, basil, vinegar, Parmesan cheese and pepper. Set aside.

3 Place bread cubes in single layer on shallow baking pan. Bake in preheated oven about 15 minutes or until lightly browned, stirring after 10 minutes. Let stand for 10 minutes.

4 In large bowl toss together bread cubes, lettuce, tomatoes, cucumber, onion and olives. Drizzle dressing over salad. Toss until coated. Let stand for 10 minutes. Toss again before serving.

Make it your own

Customize this salad by using your own favorite combination of fresh vegetables. Almost anything works well against the backdrop of crisp bread chunks in this recipe. For example:

- Replace some or all of the romaine with mixed baby greens, peppery watercress or baby spinach leaves

- In place of the cucumber try diced green, yellow or orange bell pepper

- In place of red onion, add sliced green onions or sweet yellow onion

NUTRITION FACTS PER SERVING Calories: 90; Calories from Fat: 20; **Total Fat:** 2g; **Saturated Fat:** 0g; **Trans Fat:** 0g; **Cholesterol:** 0mg; **Sodium:** 250mg; **Total Carbohydrate:** 16g; **Dietary Fiber:** 2g; **Sugars:** 4g; **Protein:** 8g

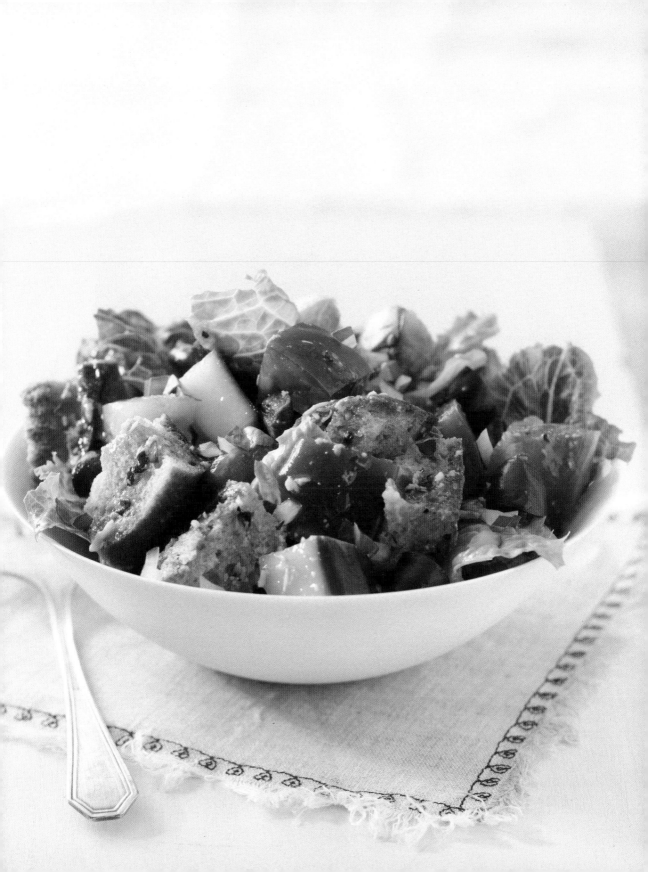

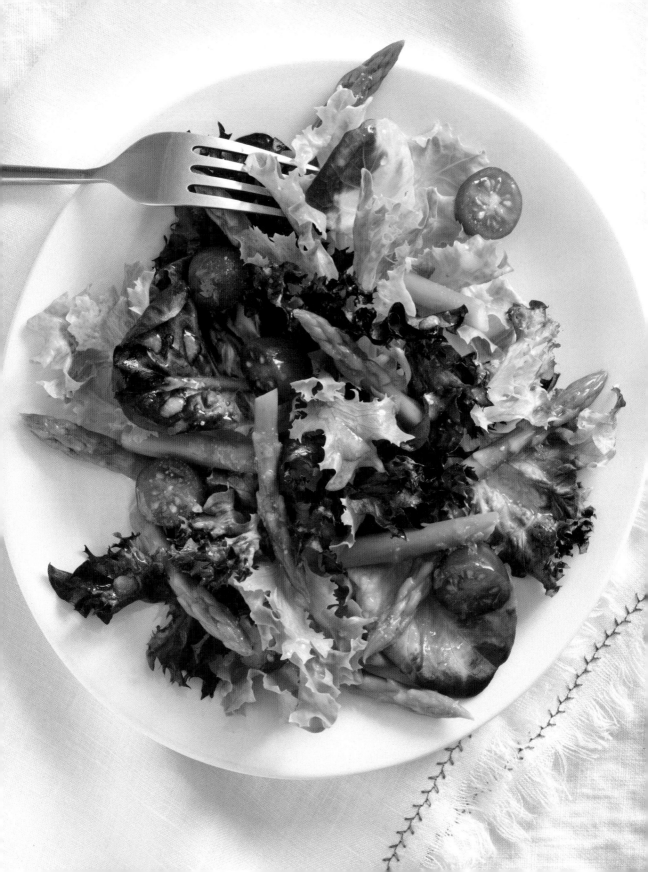

Asparagus Salad
WITH Citrus Dressing

12 ounces fresh asparagus

2 tablespoons water

¼ cup orange juice

2 teaspoons spicy
brown mustard

2 teaspoons lemon juice

2 teaspoons sugar

1 teaspoon olive oil

½ teaspoon grated
lemon zest

6 cups torn mixed
spring greens

½ cup grape tomatoes or
cherry tomatoes, halved

Just a touch of olive oil per serving brings together this tangy-spicy dressing. Try it on other microwave-steamed fresh vegetables such as sugar snap peas, broccoli or carrots.

1 Trim asparagus. Cut asparagus into 1½-inch pieces. In microwave-safe 1-quart casserole combine asparagus and water. Cover and micro-cook at high for 3 to 5 minutes or until asparagus is crisp-tender, stirring once halfway through cooking time. Drain. Rinse with cold water. Drain well. Cover with plastic wrap and refrigerate at least 45 minutes.

2 Meanwhile, in small bowl whisk together orange juice, mustard, lemon juice, sugar, oil and lemon zest. Set aside.

3 In salad bowl toss together asparagus, greens and tomatoes. Whisk orange juice mixture. Drizzle over salad. Toss until coated. Serve immediately.

NUTRITION FACTS PER SERVING Calories: 60; Calories from Fat: 15; **Total Fat:** 1.5g; **Saturated Fat:** 0g; **Trans Fat:** 0g; **Cholesterol:** 0mg; **Sodium:** 50mg; **Total Carbohydrate:** 10g; **Dietary Fiber:** 4g; **Sugars:** 4g; **Protein:** 3g

Black Bean AND Corn Dip WITH Oven-Baked Chips

1 can (15 ounces) black beans, rinsed and drained

1 cup frozen roasted whole kernel corn or whole kernel corn, thawed

1 cup seeded and finely chopped tomato

½ cup sliced green onions

¼ cup chopped fresh cilantro

3 tablespoons lime juice

1 teaspoon cumin

⅛ teaspoon garlic salt

5 ounces baked tortilla chips (about 80 chips)

Colorful and packed with robust flavor, this chunky dip makes a perfect treat to share with friends at a party or to start a casual meal, especially paired with oven-baked chips.

1 In medium bowl toss together beans, corn, tomato, onions, cilantro, lime juice, cumin and garlic salt.

2 Serve immediately or cover and refrigerate for up to 24 hours. Stir before serving. Serve with tortilla chips.

Here's to your health

Canned foods, such as the black beans used in this recipe, can be fairly high in sodium. Salt is added to enhance flavor and help preserve foods, but it can also contribute to high blood pressure. Here are three smart ways to reduce the sodium level:

Rinse before use Scientific studies have found that gently rinsing and draining canned foods before using them in a recipe can lower the sodium content.

Shop smarter More and more manufacturers are producing low-sodium or sodium-free canned goods. Read labels carefully before purchasing.

Make your own Control the sodium by cooking your own dried beans at home. For a tip on soaking the beans quickly, instead of the typical overnight soak, turn to page 58.

NUTRITION FACTS PER SERVING Calories: 60; Calories from Fat: 10; Total Fat: 1g; Saturated Fat: 0g; Trans Fat: 0g; Cholesterol: 0mg; Sodium: 110mg; Total Carbohydrate: 13g; Dietary Fiber: 2g; Sugars: 1g; Protein: 2g

Caesar Salad
WITH Creamy Dressing

SERVES 6

Croutons

Two ¾-inch-thick slices French or Italian bread

Olive oil cooking spray

1 clove garlic, peeled and halved

⅛ teaspoon salt

Dressing

¼ cup low-fat cottage cheese

1 clove garlic, minced

⅓ cup nonfat plain yogurt

3 tablespoons freshly grated Parmesan cheese

2 teaspoons lemon juice

½ teaspoon anchovy paste (optional)

⅛ teaspoon pepper

Salad

8 cups torn romaine lettuce

¼ cup freshly shaved Parmesan cheese

With creamy, nonfat yogurt and low-fat cottage cheese replacing the usual egg and oil in the dressing, no one will guess that this is a slimmed down version of the classic salad.

1 For croutons, preheat oven to 325°F. Lightly coat bread slices on both sides with cooking spray. Rub garlic clove halves over both sides of each slice. Lightly sprinkle with salt. Cut into ¾-inch pieces. Spread on 15 x 10 x 1-inch baking pan. Bake about 10 minutes or until lightly browned, stirring once or twice. Set aside.

2 For dressing, in small food processor bowl combine cottage cheese and minced garlic. Cover and process until nearly smooth. Add yogurt, grated Parmesan, lemon juice, anchovy paste (if desired) and pepper. Cover and process until combined.

3 For salad, in large salad bowl toss together lettuce and croutons. Drizzle with dressing. Toss until combined. Transfer to individual bowls or plates. Sprinkle with shaved Parmesan cheese.

NUTRITION FACTS PER SERVING Calories: 100; **Calories from Fat:** 25; **Total Fat:** 2.5g; **Saturated Fat:** 1.5g; **Trans Fat:** 0g; **Cholesterol:** 5mg; **Sodium:** 340mg; **Total Carbohydrate:** 14g; **Dietary Fiber:** 2g; **Sugars:** 2g; **Protein:** 7g

Cannellini Bean AND Spinach Soup

SERVES 8

4 ounces smoked, fully cooked, reduced-fat sausage

1 cup chopped onions

1 cup chopped carrot

1 cup thinly sliced celery

3 cloves garlic, minced

2 teaspoons vegetable oil

2 cans (15 ounces each) cannellini beans, rinsed and drained

3 cups reduced-sodium chicken broth

1 cup chopped plum tomatoes

½ teaspoon dried marjoram leaves

½ teaspoon dried thyme leaves

¼ teaspoon dried rosemary leaves

¼ teaspoon pepper

4 cups fresh baby spinach

Served by the cupful as an appetizer, this hearty soup makes a great start to an Italian-themed meal. Double the portions and serve with whole-grain bread for a satisfying main dish.

1 Halve sausage lengthwise. Cut into ¼-inch-thick slices. Set aside.

2 In nonstick Dutch oven, cook onions, carrot, celery and garlic in oil over medium heat until tender.

3 Stir in sausage slices, drained beans, broth, tomatoes, marjoram, thyme, rosemary and pepper. Bring to boiling. Reduce heat. Simmer, covered, for 30 minutes.

4 Just before serving, stir in spinach until wilted. Ladle into bowls.

Make it your own

Like so many soups, this recipe is easy to vary to your tastes and with what you have in the pantry. Try these ideas:

- Substitute diced lean fully cooked ham or smoked turkey breast for the sausage slices
- Spice it up by sautéing a pinch of crushed red pepper flakes or a little minced fresh chili pepper along with onion, carrot, celery and garlic
- Garnish each serving with a light sprinkling of freshly grated Parmesan cheese

NUTRITION FACTS PER SERVING Calories: 165; **Calories from Fat:** 45; **Total Fat:** 5g; **Saturated Fat:** 1.3g; **Trans Fat:** 0g; **Cholesterol:** 10mg; **Sodium:** 230mg; **Total Carbohydrate:** 20.5g; **Dietary Fiber:** 5.5g; **Sugars:** 3g; **Protein:** 10.5g

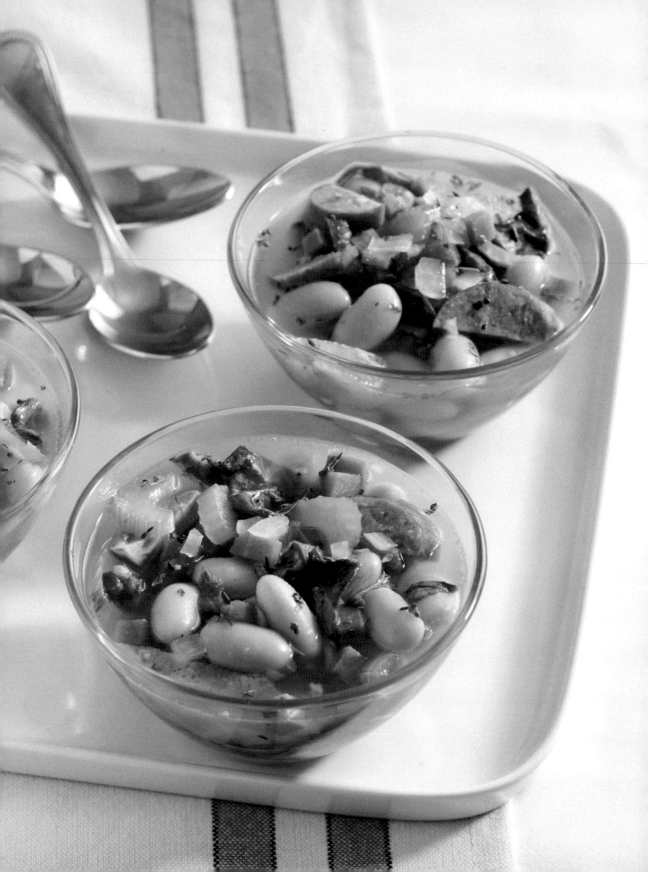

Winter Minestrone

1 cup sliced carrots

1 cup chopped onions

3 cloves garlic, minced

2 teaspoons vegetable oil

1 cup dried lentils

4 cups reduced-sodium chicken broth

1½ teaspoons dried Italian seasoning

¼ teaspoon crushed red pepper

¼ teaspoon freshly ground black pepper

4 cups coarsely chopped fresh kale

2 cans (14½ ounces each) diced tomatoes

⅓ cup grated Parmesan cheese (optional)

In this robust version of a classic Italian country-style soup, earthy-tasting lentils star with mild, cabbage-like kale, which is a source of vitamins A and C.

1 In nonstick Dutch oven, cook carrots, onions and garlic in oil over medium heat until tender.

2 Rinse and drain lentils. Stir into vegetable mixture. Stir in broth, Italian seasoning, red pepper and black pepper. Bring to boiling. Reduce heat to very low and simmer, covered, for 20 minutes. Stir in chopped kale. Return to boiling. Reduce heat. Simmer, covered, about 10 minutes or until lentils are tender.

3 Stir in tomatoes with juices. Cook, covered, for 2 to 3 minutes more or until heated through. Ladle into serving bowls. Sprinkle with Parmesan cheese, if desired.

NUTRITION FACTS PER SERVING Calories: 230; Calories from Fat: 25; **Total Fat:** 3g; **Saturated Fat:** 0g; **Trans Fat:** 0g; **Cholesterol:** 0mg; **Sodium:** 390mg; **Total Carbohydrate:** 39g; **Dietary Fiber:** 7g; **Sugars:** 9g; **Protein:** 16g

Chilled Cucumber-Mint Soup

SERVES 4

1 medium cucumber

1 cup nonfat plain yogurt

1 tablespoon lime juice

1 teaspoon honey

½ teaspoon ground cumin

⅛ teaspoon salt

¼ cup chopped fresh mint

Fresh mint leaves (optional)

Nonfat yogurt is a clever foundation for an eye-catching chilled summer soup. There's no need to wait for warm weather—you can enjoy this refreshing soup year-round.

1 Peel cucumber. Cut in half lengthwise. Scoop out seeds using teaspoon. Cut cucumber crosswise into ½-inch-thick slices.

2 In food processor bowl combine cucumber, yogurt, lime juice, honey, cumin and salt. Cover and process until smooth.

3 Transfer soup to glass mixing bowl. Stir in chopped mint. Cover with plastic wrap and refrigerate at least 1 hour. Stir before serving. Garnish individual bowls with fresh mint leaves, if desired.

Make it your own

You can turn many fresh vegetables—and even fruits—into refreshing and satisfying soups by blending them with nonfat yogurt. Try these ideas for a start:

Chilled vegetable soup After pureeing the soup in step 2, stir in 1 medium seeded and diced fresh tomato or 1 shredded carrot. Substitute fresh basil or parsley for the mint.

Icy melon soup Replace the cucumber with 1 cup peeled and chopped fresh cantaloupe or honeydew melon. Use lemon instead of lime juice and omit the salt and cumin.

Peach or nectarine soup Use 1 cup peeled and diced juicy peach or nectarine instead of the cucumber. Replace the cumin with ground cinnamon and omit the salt.

NUTRITION FACTS PER SERVING Calories: 50; **Calories from Fat:** 0; **Total Fat:** 0g; **Saturated Fat:** 0g; **Trans Fat:** 0g; **Cholesterol:** 0mg; **Sodium:** 200mg; **Total Carbohydrate:** 8g; **Dietary Fiber:** 1g; **Sugars:** 7g; **Protein:** 4g

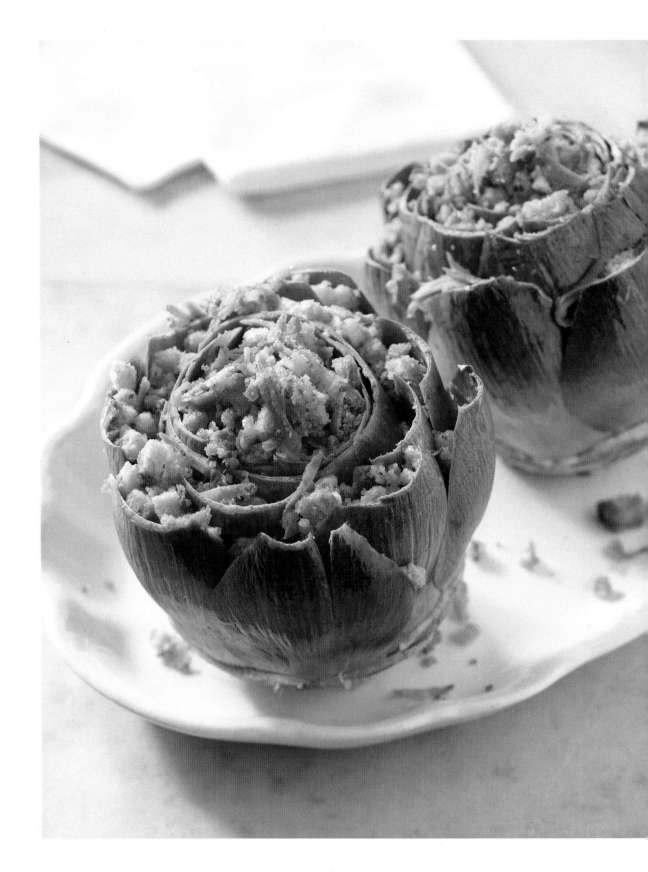

Artichokes WITH
Carrot-Cornbread Stuffing

SERVES 10

2 medium artichokes

2 tablespoons lemon juice

¾ cup water

1 cup shredded carrots

¼ cup sliced
green onions

4 teaspoons butter
or margarine

1½ cups cornbread
stuffing mix

¼ cup reduced-sodium
chicken broth

¼ teaspoon black pepper

As guests pull leaves from these artichokes, ideal for casual dining, they'll enjoy the tasty stuffing along with the nutty artichoke as they scrape off the flesh with their teeth.

1 With sharp knife, cut top 1 inch of leaves off artichokes. Remove tough outer leaves. With kitchen scissors, snip off all remaining spiky tips from leaves. Cut off stem, creating flat bottom. Brush all cut edges with lemon juice. In 2-quart, microwave-safe and oven-safe casserole, place artichokes and ¼ cup of the water. Micro-cook at high for 5 to 7 minutes or until nearly tender, turning once after 3 minutes. Drain artichokes well. Let stand upside-down on paper towels until cool enough to handle.

2 Meanwhile, in small saucepan cook carrots and onions in butter over medium-high heat until tender. Remove from heat. Stir in ¼ cup of the remaining water, stuffing mix, broth and pepper.

3 Preheat oven to 375°F.

4 Gently pull open center leaves of artichokes until you see fuzzy choke. Using melon baller or grapefruit spoon, scoop out choke. Discard. Slightly spread remaining artichoke leaves. Spoon stuffing mixture into center of each artichoke and between large leaves.

5 Return artichokes, stuffing side up, to same casserole. Pour remaining water into casserole around artichokes. Tightly cover with foil. Bake in preheated oven about 20 minutes or until wooden skewer easily pierces bottoms of artichokes. Carefully remove artichokes from dish and place on serving platter. Serve warm.

NUTRITION FACTS PER SERVING Calories: 70; **Calories from Fat:** 20; **Total Fat:** 2g; **Saturated Fat:** 1g; **Trans Fat:** 0g; **Cholesterol:** 5mg; **Sodium:** 170mg; **Total Carbohydrate:** 11g; **Dietary Fiber:** 2g; **Sugars:** 1g; **Protein:** 2g

Enlightened Guacamole

1 ripe avocado, halved,
pitted, peeled, and cut
into chunks

2 tablespoons canned
diced mild green chilies,
drained

1 teaspoon lime juice

½ teaspoon
ground cumin

¼ teaspoon garlic salt

¼ teaspoon black pepper

⅛ teaspoon
cayenne pepper

½ cup nonfat
plain yogurt

1½ ounces baked tortilla
scoops (about 24 chips)

Fat-free plain yogurt replaces the sour cream that is sometimes used in the popular avocado dip, resulting in a guacamole that has less fat but is still full of flavor.

1 In food processor bowl, combine avocado, chilies, lime juice, cumin, garlic salt, pepper, and cayenne pepper. Cover and process until mixture is smooth.

2 In medium bowl, fold together avocado mixture and yogurt.

3 Serve with tortilla chips for dipping.

Make it your own

Have fun varying this recipe to your own tastes by changing the seasonings or serving it with different dippers.

- In place of the canned chilies, mix in minced mild, medium or spicy fresh chili peppers or smoky-spicy canned chipotle chilies in adobo sauce

- Add minced sweet yellow onion, green onions or fresh chives, or some diced ripe tomato

- Stir in a little minced fresh cilantro

- Instead of baked tortilla chips, serve with cut-up vegetables such as carrots, celery or bell peppers

- Whole-grain crackers also go well with guacamole

NUTRITION FACTS PER SERVING **Calories:** 110; **Calories from Fat:** 70; **Total Fat:** 8g; **Saturated Fat:** 1g; **Trans Fat:** 0g; **Cholesterol:** 0mg; **Sodium:** 80mg; **Total Carbohydrate:** 10g; **Dietary Fiber:** 4g; **Sugars:** 1g; **Protein:** 2g

Lemon-Chive Ricotta Dip

1 cup fat-free
ricotta cheese

½ cup nonfat plain
Greek-style yogurt

⅓ cup chopped
fresh chives

1 tablespoon grated
lemon zest

½ teaspoon coarsely
ground pepper

¼ teaspoon sea salt

Celery sticks, carrot sticks
and bell pepper strips

Luscious nonfat ricotta cheese is easy to find in the dairy case of your local supermarket. Add fresh herbs and lemon zest for a terrific party dip for fresh vegetables.

1 In mixing bowl beat ricotta cheese on medium speed with electric mixer until fluffy. Add yogurt and beat until combined.

2 Stir in chives, lemon zest, pepper and salt. Cover with plastic wrap and refrigerate for 2 to 24 hours. Serve with vegetables for dipping.

NUTRITION FACTS PER SERVING Calories: 250; **Calories from Fat:** 0; **Total Fat:** 0g; **Saturated Fat:** 0g; **Trans Fat:** 0g; **Cholesterol:** 0mg; **Sodium:** 95mg; **Total Carbohydrate:** 4g; **Dietary Fiber:** 1g; **Sugars:** 3g; **Protein:** 2g

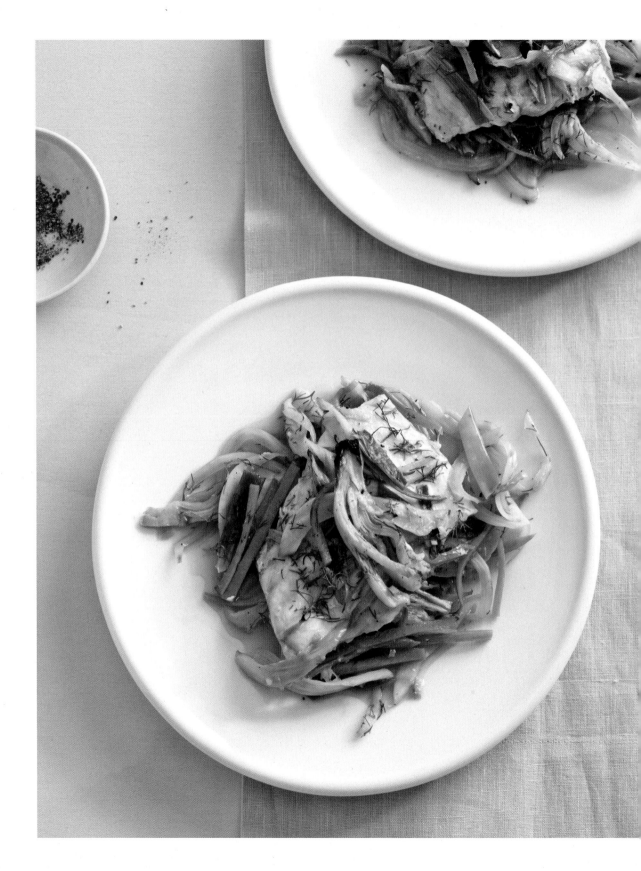

Seafood Main Dishes

Blackened Salmon-
and-Vegetable Kabobs

¾ teaspoon onion powder

¾ teaspoon garlic powder

¾ teaspoon white pepper

¾ teaspoon cayenne
pepper

¾ teaspoon black pepper

¾ teaspoon dried
thyme leaves

¼ teaspoon salt

2 large salmon steaks,
cut 1 inch thick (about
2 pounds total) or
1 pound skinless salmon
fillet, about 1 inch thick

1 tablespoon lime juice

2 medium zucchini,
halved lengthwise and
cut into ¾-inch-thick
slices (about 3½ cups)

8 cherry or grape
tomatoes

Three kinds of pepper add a spicy kick to these colorful fish-and-vegetable skewers while "blackening" them, Cajun-style. They cook in minutes on the grill or under the broiler.

1 Preheat grill or broiler. Soak 8 bamboo skewers in water to cover for 30 minutes or have ready 8 metal skewers.

2 Meanwhile, in small bowl combine onion powder, garlic powder, white pepper, cayenne pepper, black pepper, thyme and salt. Set aside.

3 Remove and discard skin and bones from salmon steaks, if using. (You should have about 1 pound salmon.) Cut fish into 1-inch pieces. In medium bowl toss fish pieces with lime juice. Sprinkle with onion powder mixture. Toss until fish is coated with spices. Drain bamboo skewers (if using). Thread fish, zucchini and tomatoes on skewers.

4 Grill kabobs on greased grill rack directly over medium-hot heat for 8 to 12 minutes or until fish flakes easily, turning frequently. Alternatively, broil on the greased rack of a broiler pan 4 to 5 inches from the heat for 8 to 12 minutes or until fish flakes easily, turning two or three times. Serve immediately.

NUTRITION FACTS PER SERVING Calories: 270; **Calories from Fat:** 140; **Total Fat:** 16g; **Saturated Fat:** 3.5g; **Trans Fat:** 0g; **Cholesterol:** 60mg; **Sodium:** 220mg; **Total Carbohydrate:** 6g; **Dietary Fiber:** 2g; **Sugars:** 3g; **Protein:** 25g

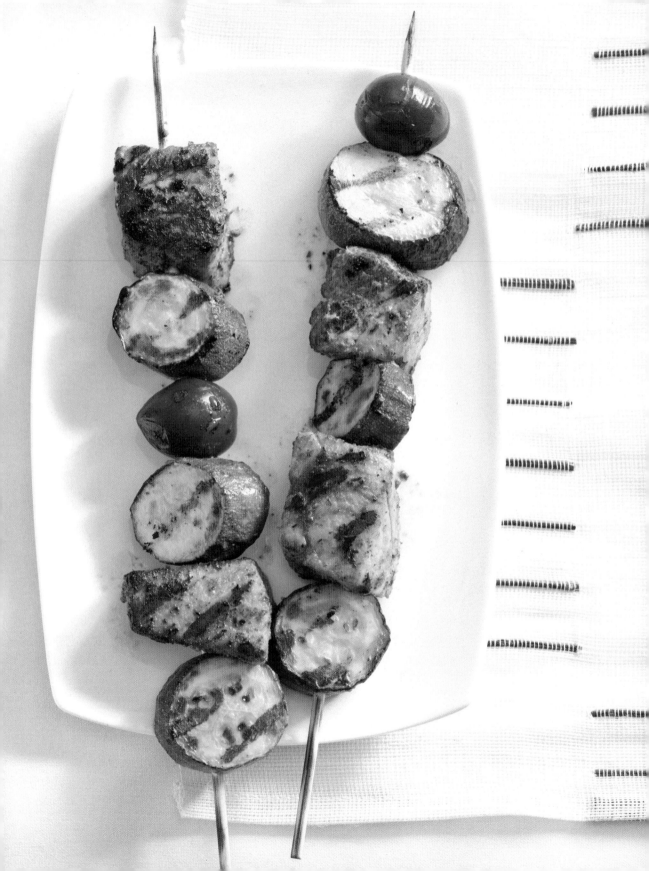

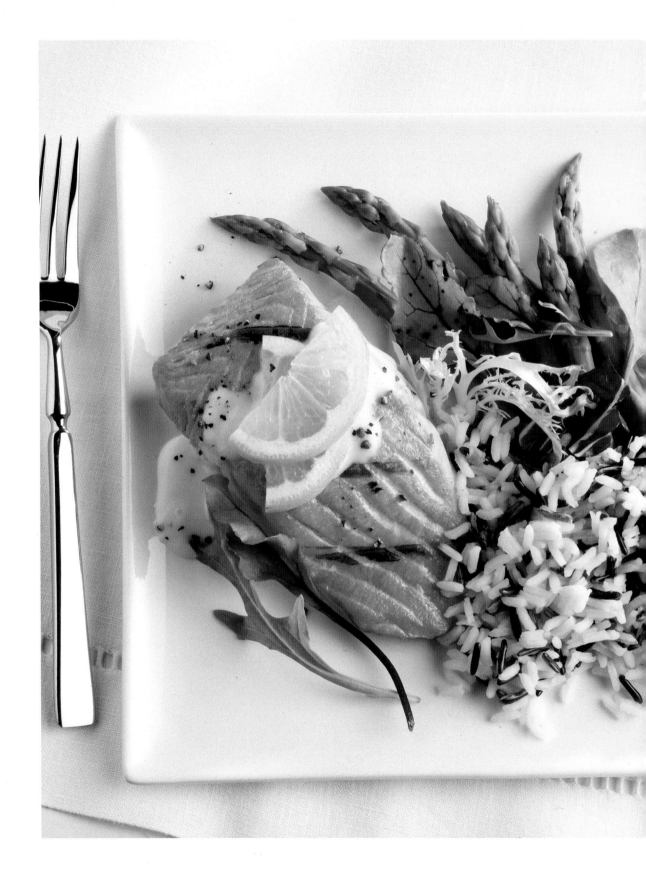

Lemon-Pepper Salmon

Four 4-ounce skinless salmon fillets, about 1 inch thick

1 teaspoon lemon-pepper seasoning salt

4 tablespoons fat-free creamy Italian dressing (optional)

4 lemon slices, cut into halves

Good-quality fresh salmon fillets are so delicious on their own that you can season them very simply. Here, a widely available seasoning blend adds bright, citrusy flavors.

1 Preheat grill or broiler.

2 Rinse salmon fillets. Pat dry with paper towels. Sprinkle seasoning salt on both sides of fillets.

3 Place salmon in well-greased grill basket and grill directly over medium heat for 8 to 12 minutes or until fish flakes with fork, turning once. Alternatively, place salmon on greased rack of broiler pan and broil 4 inches from heat for 8 to 12 minutes or until fish flakes with fork, turning once.

4 Transfer fillets to serving plates, drizzle with Italian dressing, if desired. Garnish with lemon slices.

Make it a meal

Add these delicious side dishes to each serving to create a full meal (total additional calories: 520 per serving)

- 1 cup steamed asparagus
- 1½ cups long grain and wild rice pilaf
- 1 whole-wheat dinner roll
- Tossed salad made with 1½ cups mixed greens, ¼ cup sliced cucumber, ¼ cup sliced carrots, ¼ cup halved cherry tomatoes and 2 tablespoons fat-free salad dressing

NUTRITION FACTS PER SERVING Calories: 180; Calories from Fat: 50; Total Fat: 5g; Saturated Fat: 1.5g; Trans Fat: 0g; Cholesterol: 95mg; Sodium: 120mg; Total Carbohydrate: 0g; Dietary Fiber: 0g; Sugars: 0g; Protein: 30g

Ginger AND Soy Salmon

3 tablespoons reduced-sodium soy sauce

2 tablespoons brown sugar

1 tablespoon unseasoned rice vinegar

2 teaspoons grated fresh ginger

1¼ pounds skinless salmon fillet, ¾ to 1 inch thick

Cooking spray

The simple combination of seasonings in this easy recipe adds up to very satisfying results. Use rice vinegar labeled "unseasoned," as seasoned varieties can be high in sodium.

1 In bowl stir together soy sauce, brown sugar, vinegar and ginger until sugar is dissolved. Reserve 1 tablespoon of soy mixture.

2 Cut salmon into 4 serving-size pieces. Place in resealable plastic bag. Pour in remaining soy sauce mixture. Seal bag. Place in shallow pan. Refrigerate for 1 to 2 hours, turning bag occasionally.

3 Preheat broiler.

4 Drain salmon, discarding marinade. Place on shallow baking pan lined with foil and coated with cooking spray. Broil 4 to 5 inches from heat for 8 to 12 minutes or until fish flakes with fork, turning once halfway through cooking. Transfer to serving platter. Drizzle with reserved soy sauce mixture.

NUTRITION FACTS PER SERVING **Calories:** 330; **Calories from Fat:** 170; **Total Fat:** 19g; **Saturated Fat:** 4.5g; **Trans Fat:** 0g; **Cholesterol:** 80mg; **Sodium:** 490mg; **Total Carbohydrate:** 8g; **Dietary Fiber:** 0g; **Sugars:** 7g; **Protein:** 30g

Tabbouleh-Stuffed Trout

SERVES 4

1 cup boiling water

½ cup bulgur (cracked wheat)

⅓ cup peeled and seeded finely chopped cucumber

¼ cup chopped fresh parsley

2 tablespoons sliced green onions

1 tablespoon chopped fresh mint

1 tablespoon lemon juice

2 teaspoons vegetable oil

¼ teaspoon salt

Four 8- to 10-ounce whole butterflied rainbow trout

Olive oil cooking spray

The popular Lebanese grain salad makes a satisfying and healthful stuffing for fresh fish. Ask your fish market to butterfly whole trout for you, leaving the skin intact.

1 Preheat oven to 450°F.

2 For stuffing, in medium bowl combine water and bulgur. Let stand for 20 minutes. Drain off any water. Squeeze out excess moisture. Stir in cucumber, parsley, onions, mint, lemon juice, oil and salt.

3 Place trout, skin side down, on cutting board. Spoon about ⅔ cup of the bulgur mixture inside each fish. Fold trout over stuffing. With kitchen string, gently tie each fish closed in 3 places.

4 With cooking spray, coat a shallow baking pan large enough to hold trout in a single layer. Bake in preheated oven for 10 to 15 minutes or until fish flakes easily. Transfer to individual plates and carefully cut off string before serving.

Here's to your health

The main ingredient in the tabbouleh stuffing for this recipe is bulgur. Popular in the Middle East for four millennia, it consists of kernels of whole wheat that have been steamed or parboiled, then dried and cracked into coarse pieces. Bulgur is not only a whole grain but also a source of fiber and other nutrients such as B vitamins, magnesium and iron.

NUTRITION FACTS PER SERVING Calories: 350; Calories from Fat: 90; Total Fat: 10g; Saturated Fat: 2g; Trans Fat: 0g; Cholesterol: 135mg; Sodium: 220mg; Total Carbohydrate: 14g; Dietary Fiber: 3g; Sugars: 0g; Protein: 49g

Seared Tuna Salad Niçoise

1 cup balsamic vinegar

2 teaspoons honey

½ teaspoon salt

12 ounces red-skinned new potatoes

4 teaspoons vegetable oil

½ teaspoon dried rosemary leaves

2 cloves garlic, minced

8 ounces fresh green beans, trimmed

½ medium onion, cut into slivers

1¼ pounds tuna steak or skinless tuna fillet, cut ¾ inch thick

4 cups torn romaine lettuce

1 cup grape tomatoes, halved

¼ cup pitted niçoise or Kalamata olives, chopped

In this healthful twist on a classic French dish, green beans and potatoes are roasted to intensify their flavor, and seared fresh tuna replaces the usual canned, oil-packed variety.

1 In small saucepan bring vinegar to boiling. Reduce heat. Simmer, uncovered, about 10 minutes or until vinegar is reduced by half. Stir in honey and ⅛ teaspoon of the salt. Set aside.

2 Preheat oven to 450°F.

3 Scrub potatoes. Cut any large potatoes into halves or quarters. In large bowl toss together the remaining salt, potatoes, 2 teaspoons of the oil, rosemary and garlic. In 15 x 10 x 1-inch baking pan arrange potato mixture in single layer. Bake for 10 minutes.

4 In same bowl used for potatoes toss together 1 teaspoon of the remaining oil, green beans and onion. Stir into potato mixture in baking pan. Bake about 20 minutes more or until onion begins to brown and potatoes are tender.

5 Meanwhile, cut tuna into 4 serving-size pieces. In large nonstick skillet heat remaining oil over medium-high heat. Add tuna. Cook for 5 to 10 minutes or until desired doneness, turning once.

6 In large bowl toss together potato mixture, lettuce, tomatoes and olives. Arrange on 4 serving plates. Top each with seared tuna piece. Drizzle with vinegar mixture.

NUTRITION FACTS PER SERVING Calories: 430; Calories from Fat: 120; **Total Fat:** 14g; **Saturated Fat:** 2.5g; **Trans Fat:** 0g; **Cholesterol:** 55mg; **Sodium:** 490mg; **Total Carbohydrate:** 37g; **Dietary Fiber:** 4g; **Sugars:** 18g; **Protein:** 37g

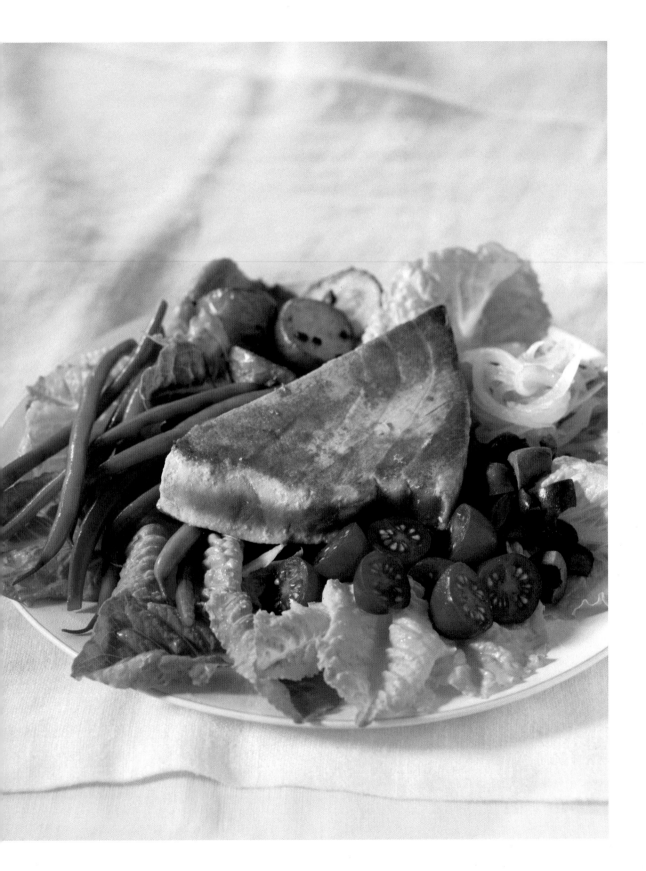

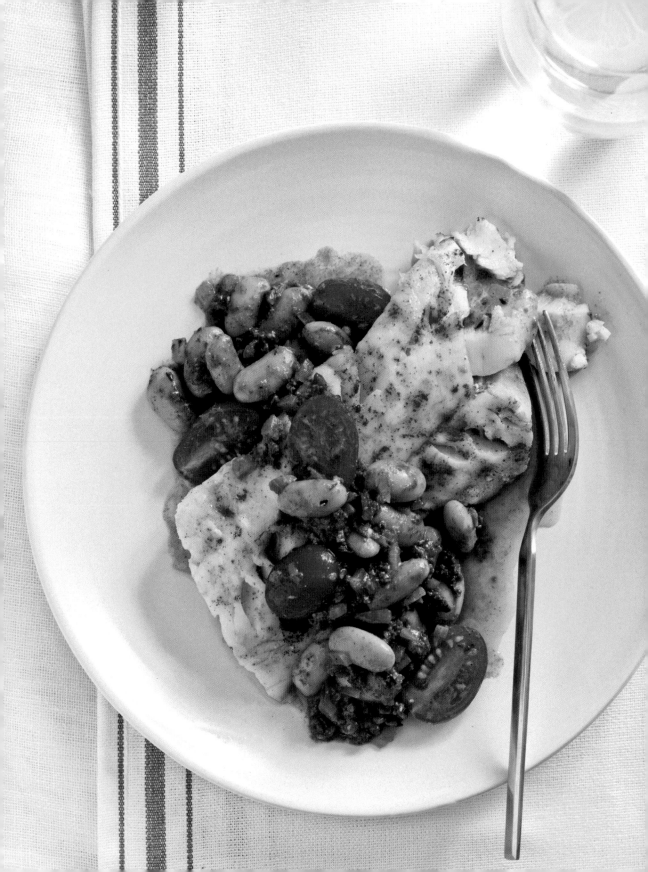

Spanish-Style Cod
WITH White Beans

3 ounces fresh chorizo
sausage or hot-style
Italian sausage, casing
slit and removed

½ cup finely
chopped onions

1 can (15 ounces) cannellini
beans, rinsed and drained

½ cup grape tomatoes or
cherry tomatoes, halved

½ teaspoon grated
orange zest

½ teaspoon dried
thyme leaves

1¼ pounds skinless cod
fillet, about ¾ inch thick

¾ teaspoon smoked
paprika or sweet paprika

Olive oil cooking spray

¼ cup reduced-sodium
chicken broth or
vegetable broth

A small piece of sausage, with much of its fat drained away, makes a big impact on the flavor of this dish. Be sure to look for fresh chorizo—the cured version won't work in this recipe.

1 Preheat oven to 425°F.

2 In small nonstick saucepan cook chorizo and onions over medium heat until onions are tender. Drain off fat. Stir in drained beans, tomatoes, orange zest and thyme.

3 Cut cod into 4 serving-size pieces. Sprinkle with paprika. Place in 13 x 9 x 2-inch baking dish coated with cooking spray. Spoon bean mixture on top of fish pieces. Pour broth into dish around fish pieces. Tightly cover with foil. Bake in preheated oven for 15 to 20 minutes or until fish flakes easily. Serve fish with bean mixture spooned over top.

Make it a meal

Add these delicious side dishes to each serving to create a full meal (total additional calories: 224 per serving)

- 2 cups mixed baby greens with 1½ tablespoons fat-free red-wine vinaigrette
- 1 medium multigrain dinner roll
- 1 cup fresh or thawed frozen mixed berries with 1 lemon wedge

NUTRITION FACTS PER SERVING Calories: 300; **Calories from Fat:** 90; **Total Fat:** 10g; **Saturated Fat:** 3.5g; **Trans Fat:** 0g; **Cholesterol:** 75mg; **Sodium:** 380mg; **Total Carbohydrate:** 17g; **Dietary Fiber:** 5g; **Sugars:** 2g; **Protein:** 33g

Crunchy Lemon Fish Fillets

1 pound fish fillets, such as fresh or frozen (thawed) cod, halibut or other mild white fish

2 cups **Kellogg's® Special K®** cereal (crushed to ¾ cup)

½ teaspoon grated lemon zest

½ teaspoon salt

¼ teaspoon dried tarragon leaves

⅛ teaspoon pepper

¼ cup chopped fresh parsley

2 egg whites

Cooking spray

2 medium lemons, thinly sliced

By coating fish fillets with a seasoned mixture of crushed **Special K** cereal and baking them, you can enjoy fried fish without the calories and fat that come from deep-frying.

1 Preheat oven to 375°F.

2 Rinse fish fillets and pat dry with paper towels. Set aside.

3 Place **Special K** cereal in shallow dish or pan. Stir in lemon zest, salt, tarragon, pepper and chopped parsley.

4 Dip fish fillets in egg whites, coating both sides. Generously coat both sides with cereal mixture, lightly pressing crumbs into fish. Place in single layer on shallow baking pan lined with foil and coated with cooking spray.

5 Bake in preheated oven about 25 minutes or until fish flakes easily. Do not cover or turn fish while baking. Serve with lemon slices.

Make it a meal

Add these delicious side dishes to each serving to create a full meal (total additional calories: 270 per serving)

- 3 ounces oven-baked frozen French fries with 1 tablespoon tomato ketchup
- 1 serving Broccoli-Pineapple Slaw (page 197)
- ½ cup lemonade mixed with ½ cup unsweetened iced tea

NUTRITION FACTS PER SERVING Calories: 170; Calories from Fat: 10; Total Fat: 1g; Saturated Fat: 0g; Trans Fat: 0g; Cholesterol: 40mg; Sodium: 530mg; Total Carbohydrate: 14g; Dietary Fiber: 2g; Sugars: 2g; Protein: 26g

Vegetable-Stuffed Swordfish

1 cup shredded carrots

⅓ cup sliced green onions

1 clove garlic

2 teaspoons butter or margarine

⅔ cup **Kellogg's® Special K®** cereal (crushed to ⅓ cup)

2 teaspoons chopped fresh marjoram or ½ teaspoon dried marjoram leaves

1½ to 1¾ pounds fresh or frozen (thawed) swordfish steaks, cut 1 inch thick

Cooking spray

Lemon wedges

Here, a mixture of carrots and green onions—plus **Special K** cereal for flavor, texture and nutrients—is stuffed inside thick, meaty swordfish steaks for a complete meal.

1 Preheat grill or broiler.

2 In small saucepan over medium heat cook carrots, onions and garlic in butter until tender. Stir in **Special K** cereal and marjoram.

3 Remove any bones from fish, if necessary. Cut into 4 serving-size portions. With a small, sharp knife cut a pocket in each portion by cutting along one side almost through to the other side.

4 Spoon carrot-cereal mixture into pockets in swordfish pieces. Secure with closed wooden toothpicks.

5 Place swordfish in well-greased grill basket and grill directly over medium heat about 12 minutes, or until fish flakes easily, turning once halfway through. Alternatively, place fish on greased rack of broiler pan and broil 4 to 5 inches from heat for about 12 minutes or until fish flakes easily, turning once halfway through.

6 Remove toothpicks. Serve with lemon wedges.

NUTRITION FACTS PER SERVING Calories: 190; Calories from Fat: 60; Total Fat: 7g; Saturated Fat: 1.5g; Trans Fat: 0g; Cholesterol: 45mg; Sodium: 170mg; Total Carbohydrate: 18g; Dietary Fiber: 1g; Sugars: 3g; Protein: 25g

Greek-Style Halibut

1¼ pounds skinless halibut or other mild, white fish fillet, ¾ to 1 inch thick

¼ teaspoon salt

1 teaspoon vegetable oil

½ medium onion, thinly sliced

2 cloves garlic, minced

¼ cup reduced-sodium chicken broth or vegetable broth

4 medium tomatoes, peeled, seeded and chopped (about 2½ cups)

¼ cup chopped, pitted black Cerignola olives or Kalamata olives

½ teaspoon dried oregano leaves

¼ teaspoon crushed red pepper

¼ cup crumbled reduced-fat feta cheese

Fresh tomatoes, black olives, oregano and feta cheese lend Greek-influenced flavors to a quick, low-fat pan sauce for fish fillets. It's a perfect main dish for warm-weather dining.

1 Cut halibut into 4 serving-size pieces. Lightly sprinkle with salt.

2 In large nonstick skillet heat oil over medium-high heat. Add halibut pieces. Quickly sear for 3 to 4 minutes or until beginning to brown, turning once. Remove from skillet. Keep warm.

3 Add onion and garlic to same skillet. Stir in 2 tablespoons of the broth. Cook, covered, over medium heat until onion is tender. Stir in remaining broth, tomatoes, olives, oregano and red pepper. Bring to boiling. Return halibut to skillet. Cook, covered, over medium heat for 3 to 5 minutes more or until fish flakes easily with fork.

4 Transfer fish to serving platter. Spoon tomato mixture on fish. Sprinkle feta cheese on top.

NUTRITION FACTS PER SERVING **Calories:** 240; **Calories from Fat:** 70; **Total Fat:** 8g; **Saturated Fat:** 1.5g; **Trans Fat:** 0g; **Cholesterol:** 50mg; **Sodium:** 440mg; **Total Carbohydrate:** 10g; **Dietary Fiber:** 2g; **Sugars:** 5g; **Protein:** 33g

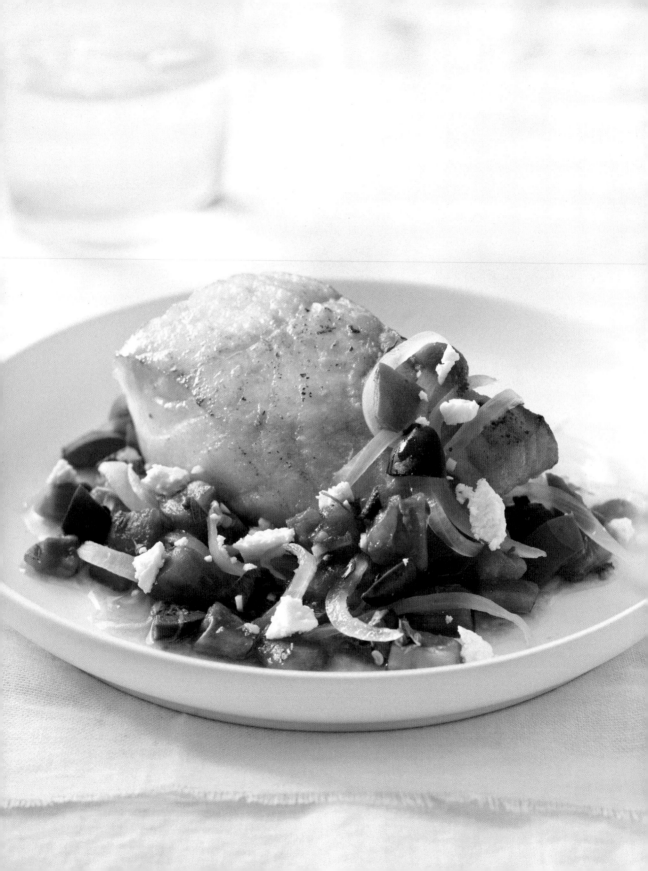

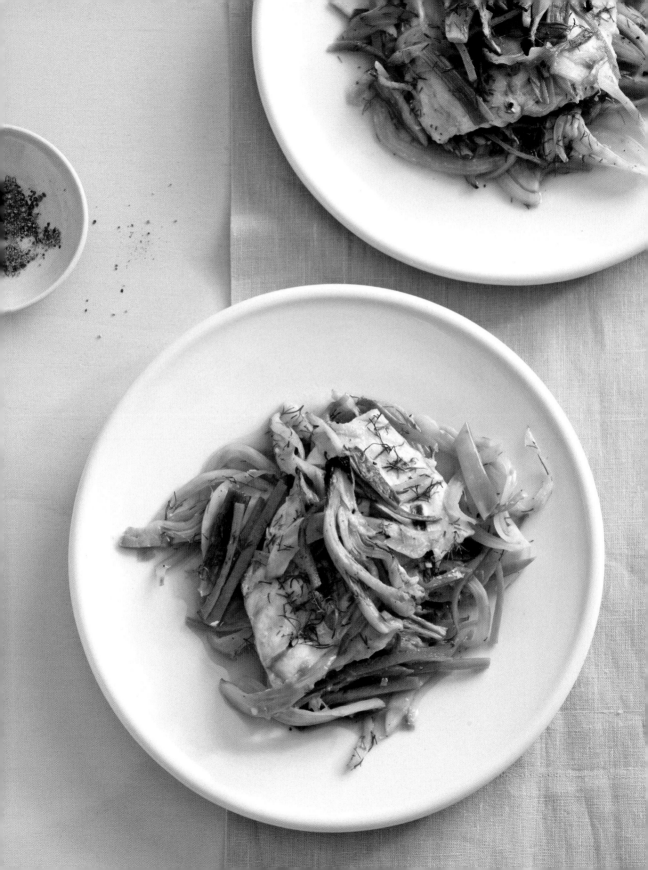

Baked Snapper
WITH Fennel AND Dill

2 fennel bulbs, trimmed and thinly sliced (about 2½ cups)

2 cloves garlic, minced

2 teaspoons vegetable oil

1 cup matchstick-cut carrots

4 green onions, cut into 1-inch pieces

3 tablespoons chopped fresh dill

1 teaspoon grated lemon zest

¼ teaspoon salt

¼ teaspoon pepper

Cooking spray

1 pound skinless snapper fillets, about ½ inch thick

¼ cup reduced-sodium chicken broth

Fresh fennel, dill and lemon harmonize beautifully in this easy main dish. Baking in this manner helps keep thin, delicate fish fillets intact for a pretty presentation.

1 Preheat oven to 450°F.

2 Meanwhile, in large nonstick skillet cook fennel and garlic in oil over medium heat for 7 to 9 minutes or until fennel is tender. Stir in carrots, green onions, dill, lemon zest, salt and pepper.

3 Set aside 1 cup of the vegetable mixture. Spoon remaining vegetable mixture into 12 x 8 x 2-inch baking dish coated with cooking spray. Cut fish into 4 serving-size pieces. Place on top of vegetables. Sprinkle reserved vegetable mixture over fish. Drizzle with broth.

4 Bake, uncovered, in preheated oven for 15 to 20 minutes or until fish flakes easily with fork. Serve immediately.

Make it your own

You can easily use this recipe as a base for improvising your own baked fish dishes. Try these ideas:

- Vary the vegetables, substituting any combination of sliced yellow onions, parsnips and baby turnips
- Use different mild fresh herbs, such as parsley, basil, chives, chervil or tarragon
- Substitute other delicate, thin fish fillets, including sole, flounder or halibut

NUTRITION FACTS PER SERVING Calories: 170; **Calories from Fat:** 35; **Total Fat:** 4g; **Saturated Fat:** 0.5g; **Trans Fat:** 0g; **Cholesterol:** 40mg; **Sodium:** 280mg; **Total Carbohydrate:** 9g; **Dietary Fiber:** 3g; **Sugars:** 3g; **Protein:** 25g

Mustard-Topped Halibut in Parchment

SERVES 2

¾ cup julienne-cut carrots

2 tablespoons water

8 ounces skinless halibut fillet, about ½ inch thick

1 tablespoon spicy brown mustard

¼ teaspoon dried basil leaves

⅛ teaspoon pepper

⅛ teaspoon garlic powder

½ small zucchini, sliced ¼ inch thick (about ⅔ cup)

1 teaspoon chopped fresh chives

Baking seasoned fish fillets and vegetables inside easy-to-assemble parcels of parchment paper seals in moisture and flavor and makes an elegant presentation.

1 Preheat oven to 450°F.

2 In microwave-safe 2-cup casserole combine carrots and water. Cover and micro-cook at high for 1 minute. Drain well.

3 Cut halibut into 2 serving-size portions. Cut two 15 x 12-inch pieces of parchment paper into heart shapes that are about 6 inches longer and 2 inches wider than fish portions. Place one fish portion on right side of each parchment heart.

4 In small bowl stir together mustard, basil, pepper and garlic powder. Spread mustard mixture over fish portions. Top with carrots and zucchini. Sprinkle with chives.

5 Fold left side of each parchment heart over fish, forming half-heart shapes. Starting at top of heart halves, seal by folding edges together in small pleats. Twist bottom tips to secure closed. Place on baking sheet. Bake in preheated oven for 15 to 18 minutes or until paper turns light brown and fish flakes easily.

6 To serve, transfer parcels to serving plates. With tip of sharp knife or kitchen scissors carefully cut large X on top of each, avoiding hot steam. Carefully pull back paper. Serve immediately.

NUTRITION FACTS PER SERVING Calories: 160; Calories from Fat: 30; Total Fat: 3.5g; Saturated Fat: 1g; Trans Fat: 0g; Cholesterol: 80mg; Sodium: 200mg; Total Carbohydrate: 7g; Dietary Fiber: 2g; Sugars: 3g; Protein: 24g

New Orleans–Style Pecan-Crusted Fish

SERVES 4

3¾ cups **Kellogg's®
Special K®** cereal
(crushed to 1¼ cups)

⅓ cup finely chopped
pecans, toasted

1 teaspoon chili powder

½ teaspoon paprika

¼ teaspoon salt

¼ teaspoon
cayenne pepper

⅛ teaspoon
garlic powder

½ cup low-fat buttermilk

⅓ cup all-purpose flour

1¼ pounds skinless tilapia
fillets, about ¾ inch thick

Olive oil cooking spray

Fish fillets with a delicious, crispy crust can still be lean and healthful. This oven-baked version features a spicy coating of **Special K** cereal mixed with toasted pecan pieces.

1 Preheat oven to 450°F.

2 In shallow dish combine **Special K** cereal, pecans, chili powder, paprika, salt, cayenne pepper and garlic powder. Set aside.

3 Pour buttermilk into another shallow dish. Spread flour in even layer on sheet of wax paper.

4 Cut tilapia into 4 serving-size pieces, if necessary. Lightly coat fish with flour. Dip into buttermilk, coating both sides. Generously coat both sides with cereal mixture, lightly pressing crumbs into fish. Place in single layer on baking sheet lined with foil and coated with cooking spray. Lightly coat tops of fish pieces with additional cooking spray.

5 Bake, uncovered, in preheated oven about 8 minutes or until lightly browned. Carefully turn fish with a spatula. Bake for 4 to 7 minutes more or until fish flakes easily. Serve immediately.

NUTRITION FACTS PER SERVING Calories: 360; Calories from Fat: 90; **Total Fat:** 10g; **Saturated Fat:** 2g; **Trans Fat:** 0g; **Cholesterol:** 70mg; **Sodium:** 460mg; **Total Carbohydrate:** 31g; **Dietary Fiber:** 2g; **Sugars:** 6g; **Protein:** 38g

Sautéed Shrimp Tacos

1 pound fresh or frozen medium shrimp

1 large mango, peeled, seeded and finely chopped

½ cup seeded and chopped tomato

¼ cup sliced green onions

1 jalapeño chili, seeded and finely chopped

1 tablespoon lime juice

1 teaspoon Caribbean jerk seasoning

2 teaspoons vegetable oil

3 cups shredded fresh spinach

Eight 6-inch whole-wheat, spinach or flour tortillas, warmed

Bold, but not too spicy, this recipe uses Jamaican-style jerk spices. Widely available, the spice blend generally includes chilies, thyme, cinnamon, ginger, allspice and cloves.

1 Thaw shrimp, if frozen. Peel and devein shrimp, if necessary. Cover and refrigerate until needed.

2 In medium bowl stir together mango, tomato, green onions, jalapeño chili and lime juice. Set aside.

3 Toss shrimp with jerk seasoning. In large nonstick skillet heat 1 teaspoon of the oil medium-high heat. Add half of the shrimp. Cook and stir for 2 to 3 minutes or until shrimp turn opaque. Remove from skillet. Repeat with remaining 1 teaspoon oil and remaining shrimp.

4 Serve shrimp, spinach and mango mixture in tortillas.

Make it a meal

Add these delicious sides to each serving to create a full meal (total additional calories: 311 per serving)

- 1 serving Enlightened Guacamole (page 94)
- ½ cup canned fat-free refried beans
- 1 cup spicy tomato-vegetable juice
- 1 cup fresh papaya cubes with 1 lime wedge

NUTRITION FACTS PER SERVING Calories: 470; Calories from Fat: 90; Total Fat: 11g; Saturated Fat: 0.5g; Trans Fat: 0g; Cholesterol: 170mg; Sodium: 600mg; Total Carbohydrate: 56g; Dietary Fiber: 6g; Sugars: 11g; Protein: 32g

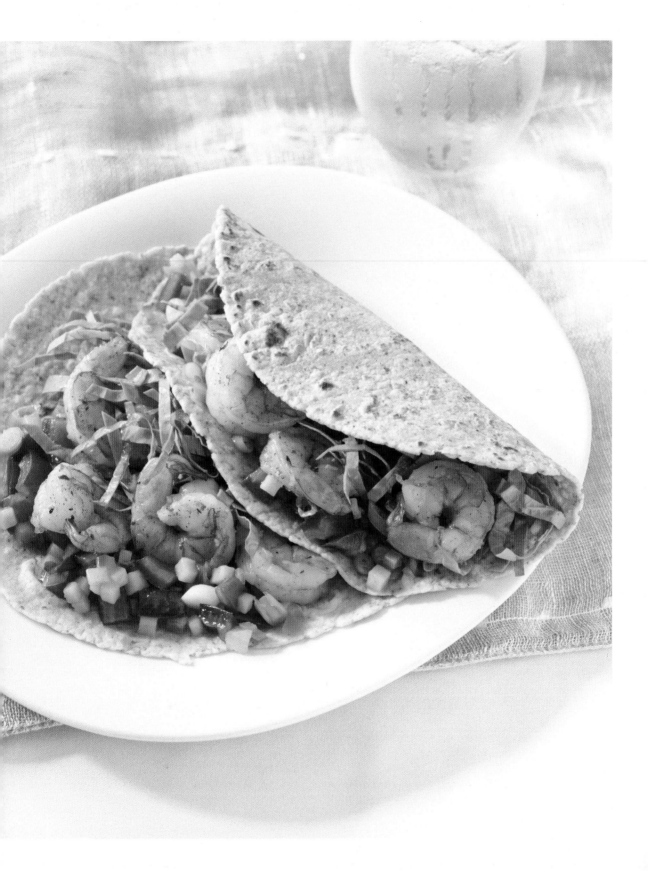

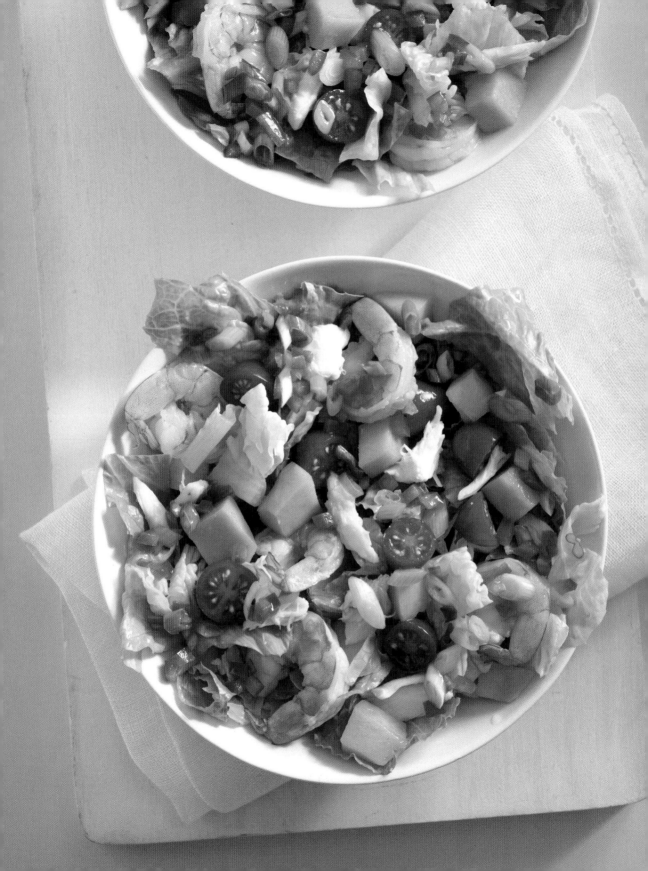

Crab AND Shrimp Salad

½ cup lime juice

¼ cup finely chopped
red bell pepper

¼ cup sliced
green onions

3 tablespoons olive oil

1½ teaspoons sugar

¼ teaspoon garlic salt

6 ounces cooked,
peeled and deveined
medium shrimp

6 ounces cooked
lump crabmeat

6 cups torn romaine
lettuce

1½ cups coarsely
chopped fresh mango
(about 2 medium)

1 cup grape tomatoes or
cherry tomatoes, halved

This lively combination of seafood, vegetables and tropical fruit tossed with a zesty dressing shows how satisfying a healthy salad can be when served as a dinnertime main dish.

1 In small bowl whisk together lime juice, bell pepper, green onions, olive oil, 1 teaspoon of the sugar and salt. Cover and refrigerate ⅓ cup of the mixture to use for dressing.

2 In large resealable plastic bag combine the remaining lime juice mixture, shrimp and crabmeat. Seal bag. Refrigerate for 2 to 3 hours, turning bag occasionally.

3 Drain shrimp and crabmeat, discarding marinade. In large salad bowl toss together marinated shrimp, crabmeat, lettuce, mango and tomatoes. Whisk remaining ½ teaspoon sugar into reserved dressing. Drizzle over salad. Toss until coated. Serve immediately.

Make it your own

Shellfish like the shrimp and crab in this recipe are often described as "sweet" because of their mild, pleasant flavor. That helps them go well with many kinds of juicy fruit. In place of the fresh mango in this recipe, you could try diced papaya or pineapple, or nontropical fruit like halved seedless grapes or diced nectarine or peach. You can also substitute small cooked and chilled bay scallops for some of the shrimp or crabmeat.

NUTRITION FACTS PER SERVING Calories: 260; Calories from Fat: 110; **Total Fat:** 12g; **Saturated Fat:** 1.5g; **Trans Fat:** 0g; **Cholesterol:** 115mg; **Sodium:** 350mg; **Total Carbohydrate:** 20g; **Dietary Fiber:** 2g; **Sugars:** 14g; **Protein:** 21g

Kung Pao Shrimp Stir-Fry

12 ounces peeled and
deveined medium shrimp

2 teaspoons cornstarch

¼ teaspoon white pepper

3 tablespoons rice vinegar

2 tablespoons
hoisin sauce

2 tablespoons reduced-
sodium soy sauce

1 teaspoon sugar

½ teaspoon crushed
red pepper

2 teaspoons vegetable oil

½ medium onion, cut
into ½-inch pieces

2 teaspoons grated
fresh ginger

1 small jalapeño chili,
seeded and finely
chopped

1 clove garlic, minced

4 cups broccoli florets

½ cup canned sliced
bamboo shoots, drained

2 cups hot cooked
brown rice

¼ cup dry-roasted
unsalted peanuts

Here's a version of a popular Chinese takeout dish that's been re-imagined for the health-minded eater. The key is a sweet-sour-spicy sauce that tops tender shrimp and broccoli.

1 In medium bowl toss together shrimp, cornstarch and white pepper. Let stand for 15 minutes.

2 Meanwhile, in small bowl stir together rice vinegar, hoisin sauce, soy sauce, sugar and crushed red pepper. Set aside.

3 Heat 1 teaspoon of the oil in nonstick wok or large nonstick skillet over high heat. Add onion. Stir-fry for 2 minutes. Add ginger, jalapeño chili and garlic. Stir-fry for 2 minutes. Add broccoli and bamboo shoots. Stir-fry for 2 to 3 minutes or until vegetables are crisp-tender. Remove from wok.

4 Add remaining oil to wok. Stir-fry shrimp mixture for 1 to 3 minutes or until shrimp are opaque. Stir vinegar mixture. Add to wok. Return vegetables to wok. Cook and stir until heated through. Serve over rice. Sprinkle with peanuts.

NUTRITION FACTS PER SERVING **Calories:** 340; **Calories from Fat:** 90; **Total Fat:** 10g; **Saturated Fat:** 1.5g; **Trans Fat:** 0g; **Cholesterol:** 130mg; **Sodium:** 740mg; **Total Carbohydrate:** 41g; **Dietary Fiber:** 6g; **Sugars:** 8g; **Protein:** 25g

Thai-Style Scallops with Cabbage

SERVES 4

2 teaspoons vegetable oil

½ cup sliced green onions

2 cloves garlic, minced

1 to 2 fresh red Thai bird chilies, or other small, fresh, spicy or mild chilies, seeded and thinly sliced

12 ounces bay scallops

3 cups thinly sliced green cabbage

2 cups cooked brown rice

1 cup matchstick-cut carrots

2 tablespoons reduced-sodium soy sauce

1 tablespoon lime juice

2 teaspoons fish sauce

¼ cup chopped fresh Thai basil or chopped fresh basil

1 tablespoon chopped fresh mint

Lively Thai seasonings and fresh herbs bring contemporary appeal to this dish. Look for bottled fish sauce in ethnic markets or the Asian foods aisle of your supermarket.

1 Heat 1 teaspoon of the oil in nonstick wok or large nonstick skillet over high heat. Add green onions, garlic and chilies. Stir-fry for 1 minute. Add scallops. Stir-fry for 2 to 4 minutes or until scallops are opaque. Remove from wok.

2 Add remaining oil to wok or skillet. Add cabbage, rice, carrots, soy sauce, lime juice and fish sauce. Stir-fry about 2 minutes or until heated through. Add basil and mint. Stir-fry about 30 seconds more or until herbs begin to wilt. Stir in scallop mixture. Heat through. Serve immediately.

Make it a meal

Add these delicious side dishes to each serving to create a full meal (total additional calories: 345 per serving)

- 1 cup steamed jasmine rice
- Frozen Yogurt and Berry Sundae (page 231)
- Unsweetened regular or passion fruit iced tea

NUTRITION FACTS PER SERVING **Calories:** 250; **Calories from Fat:** 35; **Total Fat:** 4g; **Saturated Fat:** 0g; **Trans Fat:** 0g; **Cholesterol:** 30mg; **Sodium:** 710mg; **Total Carbohydrate:** 35g; **Dietary Fiber:** 5g; **Sugars:** 6g; **Protein:** 19g

Crispy Baked Crab Cakes
with Spicy Rémoulade

SERVES 4

½ cup nonfat plain Greek-style yogurt

3 tablespoons reduced-fat mayonnaise

2 teaspoons lime juice

½ teaspoon ground cumin

¼ teaspoon cayenne pepper

⅛ teaspoon garlic powder

¼ cup finely chopped celery

¼ cup finely chopped green onions

¼ cup finely chopped red bell pepper

2 tablespoons refrigerated fat-free egg product

½ teaspoon grated lime zest

¼ teaspoon garlic salt

3 cups **Kellogg's® Special K®** cereal (crushed to 1 cup)

2 cans (4¼ ounces each) lump crabmeat, well drained

Olive oil cooking spray

Old-fashioned crab cakes take a healthy turn when coated with **Special K** cereal and baked instead of fried. The bold sauce is a light version of the traditional accompaniment.

1 Preheat oven to 425°F.

2 In small bowl stir together ¼ cup of the yogurt, mayonnaise, lime juice, cumin, ⅛ teaspoon of the cayenne pepper and garlic powder. Cover and refrigerate until needed.

3 In large bowl stir together remaining yogurt, remaining cayenne pepper, celery, onions, bell pepper, egg product, lime zest and garlic salt. Stir in ⅓ cup of the **Special K** cereal. Add crabmeat. Mix well. Place remaining cereal in shallow dish.

4 Shape crab mixture into eight 1-inch-thick patties. Dip patties into cereal, coating both sides and lightly pressing crumbs into patties. Place on baking sheet coated with cooking spray. Lightly coat tops of crabcake patties with additional cooking spray. Bake in preheated oven about 10 minutes or until lightly browned. Turn patties over and bake about 10 minutes more, or until lightly browned. Serve with reserved yogurt mixture.

NUTRITION FACTS PER SERVING Calories: 210; Calories from Fat: 45; Total Fat: 5g; Saturated Fat: 1g; Trans Fat: 0g; Cholesterol: 45mg; Sodium: 570mg; Total Carbohydrate: 20g; Dietary Fiber: 1g; Sugars: 5g; Protein: 22g

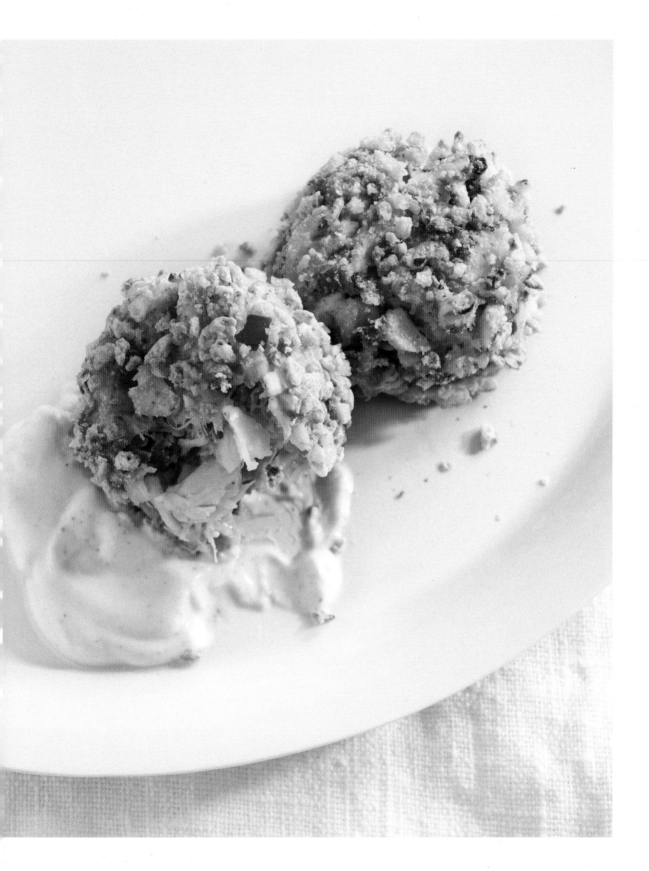

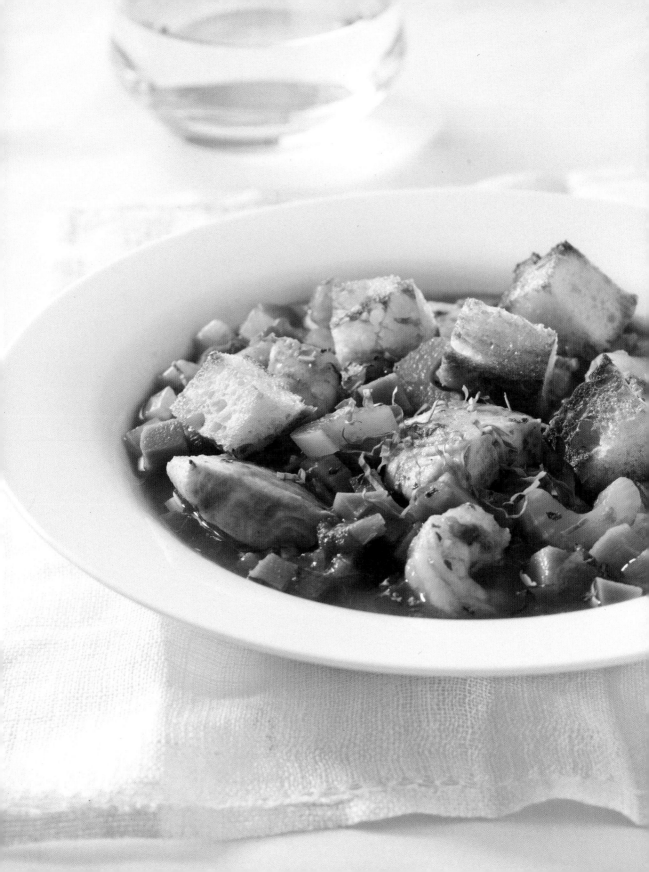

Quick Bouillabaisse
with Garlic Croutons

SERVES 4

Two 1-inch-thick slices
French bread

Olive oil cooking spray

1 clove garlic, peeled
and halved

¼ teaspoon salt

8 ounces fresh or frozen
skinless tilapia fillets

8 ounces fresh or frozen
medium shrimp in shells

1 cup chopped carrot

¾ cup chopped onions

½ cup sliced celery

2 cloves garlic, minced

2 teaspoons vegetable oil

1 can (14½ ounces)
no-added-salt diced
tomatoes

1¼ cups reduced-sodium
chicken broth

1 can (8 ounces)
tomato sauce

½ teaspoon dried
basil leaves

½ teaspoon turmeric

¼ teaspoon fennel
seeds, crushed

⅛ teaspoon crushed
red pepper

Slivered fresh basil
(optional)

This easy, healthful version of a traditional French seafood soup is ready in less than an hour. Feel free to substitute other kinds of fish or shellfish for those called for here.

1 For croutons, preheat oven to 325°F. Lightly coat bread slices on both sides with cooking spray. Rub garlic clove halves over both sides of each slice. Lightly sprinkle with salt. Cut into ¾-inch pieces. Spread on 15 x 10 x 1-inch baking pan. Bake about 10 minutes or until lightly browned, stirring once or twice. Set aside.

2 Meanwhile, thaw fish and shrimp, if frozen. Cut fish into 1-inch pieces. Peel and devein shrimp, if necessary. Cover and refrigerate.

3 In nonstick Dutch oven cook carrot, onions, celery and minced garlic in oil over medium heat until tender, stirring occasionally. Stir in undrained tomatoes, broth, tomato sauce, basil, turmeric, fennel seeds and red pepper. Bring to boiling. Reduce heat. Simmer, covered, for 20 minutes.

4 Gently stir in fish pieces and shrimp. Return to boiling. Reduce heat. Simmer, covered, for 2 to 4 minutes or until fish flakes easily and shrimp turn opaque. Ladle into serving bowls. Serve topped with croutons and fresh basil (if desired).

NUTRITION FACTS PER SERVING Calories: 270; **Calories from Fat:** 45; **Total Fat:** 5g; **Saturated Fat:** 1g; **Trans Fat:** 0g; **Cholesterol:** 115mg; **Sodium:** 430mg; **Total Carbohydrate:** 26g; **Dietary Fiber:** 4g; **Sugars:** 9g; **Protein:** 29g

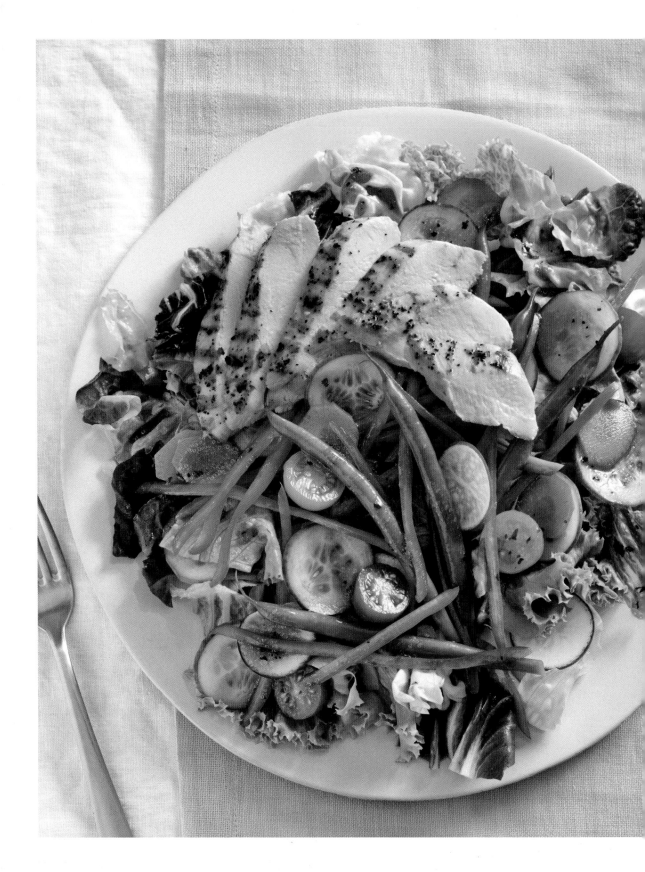

Poultry Main Dishes

Chicken AND Red Chile Enchiladas

2 cups shredded, rotisserie-roasted chicken breast

1 package (10 ounces) frozen chopped spinach, thawed and well drained

8 ounces reduced-fat sour cream

½ cup nonfat plain yogurt

2 tablespoons all-purpose flour

1 teaspoon ground cumin

2 cloves garlic, minced

⅓ cup nonfat milk

⅓ cup sliced green onions

2 red or green jalapeño chilies, seeded, deveined and finely chopped

⅛ teaspoon salt

Six (6- to 7-inch) whole-wheat tortillas or spinach tortillas

Cooking spray

½ cup shredded reduced-fat sharp cheddar cheese

¾ cup tomato salsa

Using cooked rotisserie chicken and frozen spinach make it easy to put together tasty, filling enchiladas. Add a green salad and beans or rice pilaf to complete the meal.

1 Preheat oven to 350°F.

2 In large bowl toss together chicken and spinach. In bowl stir together sour cream, yogurt, flour, cumin and garlic. Gradually stir in milk, onions and jalapeño chilies. Stir half of sour cream mixture into chicken mixture. Stir salt into remaining sour cream mixture.

3 Spoon chicken mixture down one edge of each tortilla. Roll up. Place, seam side down, in a 12 x 8 x 2-inch baking dish coated with cooking spray. Spread sour cream mixture over top.

4 Bake in preheated oven, uncovered, for 25 minutes. Sprinkle with cheese. Continue baking about 5 minutes or until heated through and cheese has melted. Let stand for 5 minutes. Serve with salsa.

Make it your own

Enchiladas are easy to vary using a variety of healthful fillings. Try these ideas for a start:

- Replace the chicken with cooked leftover turkey breast or lean, well-trimmed cooked beef, pork or lamb
- In place of the spinach, use any other chopped cooked vegetables such as broccoli, kale or green beans
- Swap out other kinds of reduced-fat cheese such as Monterey jack, pepper jack or mozzarella

NUTRITION FACTS PER SERVING Calories: 310; **Calories from Fat:** 90; **Total Fat:** 10g; **Saturated Fat:** 4g; **Trans Fat:** 0g; **Cholesterol:** 40mg; **Sodium:** 730mg; **Total Carbohydrate:** 34g; **Dietary Fiber:** 3g; **Sugars:** 4g; **Protein:** 20g

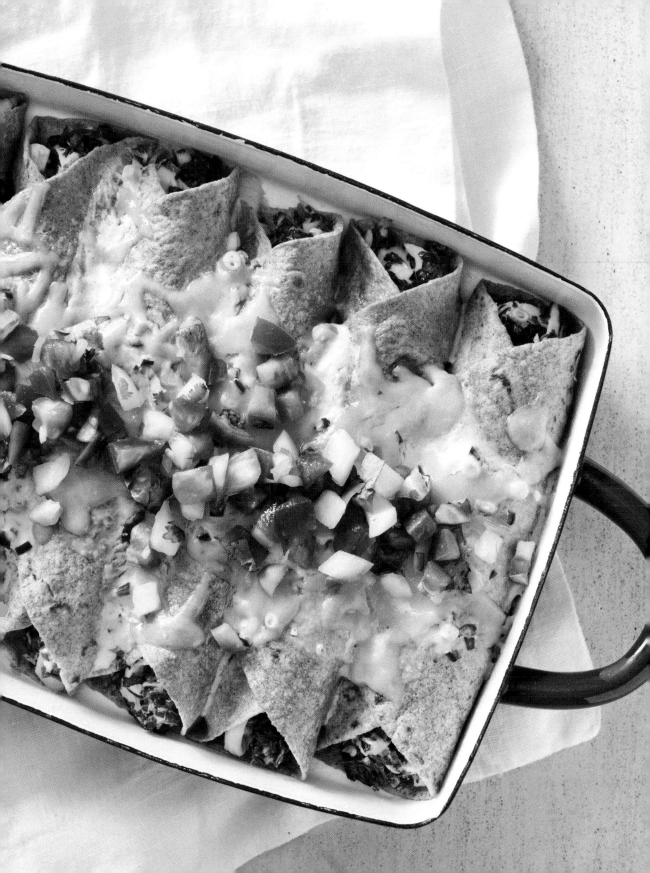

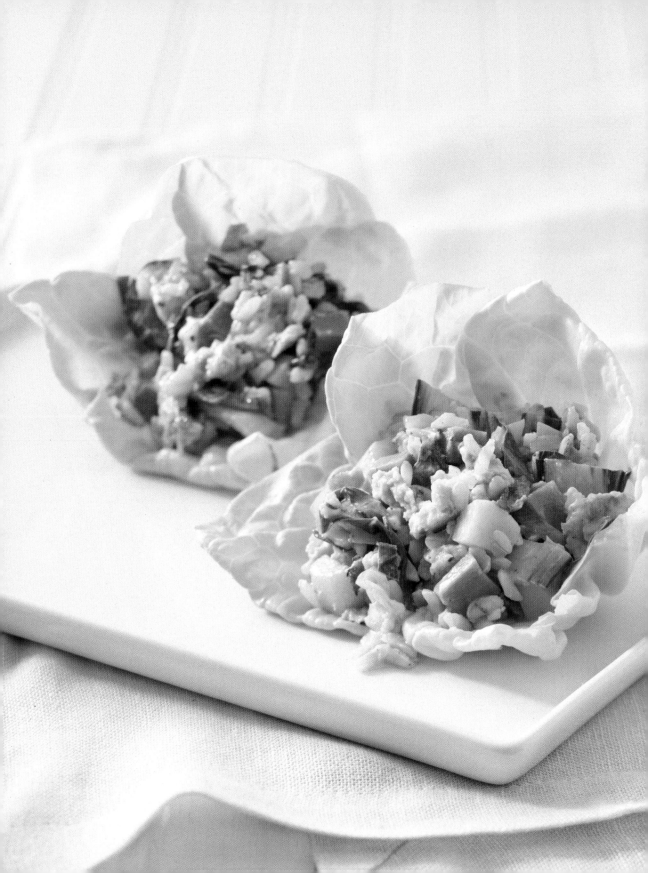

Thai-Style Chicken IN Lettuce Cups

SERVES 4

3 tablespoons
orange juice

2 tablespoons creamy
peanut butter

2 tablespoons reduced-
sodium soy sauce

1 tablespoon unseasoned
rice vinegar

2 teaspoons grated
fresh ginger

8 ounces ground
chicken breast

2 cloves garlic, minced

2 cups thinly sliced
bok choy

1½ cups cooked
brown rice

½ cup coarsely
chopped carrot

½ cup sliced
green onions

⅓ cup chopped water
chestnuts, drained

¼ teaspoon crushed
red pepper

12 medium Bibb or
Boston lettuce leaves

The salty, tangy and spicy flavors of Thai cooking help create a satisfying meal. Peanut butter adds a touch of richness to a lean chicken filling in these Asian-style, lettuce-leaf tacos.

1 In small food processor work bowl or blender container combine orange juice, peanut butter, soy sauce, vinegar and ginger. Cover and process until nearly smooth. Set aside.

2 In large nonstick skillet cook chicken and garlic over medium-high heat, breaking up chicken with a wooden spoon, for 3 to 5 minutes or until chicken is no longer pink. Drain off any fat. Stir in bok choy, rice, carrot, green onions, water chestnuts and red pepper. Stir in orange juice mixture. Reduce heat to medium. Cover and cook for 2 minutes.

3 Place lettuce on serving platter. Spoon chicken into leaves. Wrap lettuce around chicken, securing with wooden picks (if desired).

Make it a meal

Add these delicious side dishes to each serving to create a full meal (total additional calories: 305 per serving)

- Asian-Style Braised Baby Bok Choy (page 205)
- Gingered Cantaloupe with Raspberries (page 77)
- Iced or hot green tea

NUTRITION FACTS PER SERVING **Calories:** 230; **Calories from Fat:** 60; **Total Fat:** 6g; **Saturated Fat:** 1.5g; **Trans Fat:** 0g; **Cholesterol:** 35mg; **Sodium:** 440mg; **Total Carbohydrate:** 27g; **Dietary Fiber:** 4g; **Sugars:** 4g; **Protein:** 18g

Apple-Cherry Poached Chicken

¾ cup plus ⅓ cup apple juice

¾ teaspoon instant chicken bouillon granules

1 clove garlic, minced

4 small boneless, skinless chicken breast halves (about 16 ounces total)

1 medium cooking apple, cored and thinly sliced

½ cup dried tart cherries

2 teaspoons cornstarch

½ teaspoon cinnamon

⅛ teaspoon cayenne pepper

Poaching is one of the healthiest ways to cook. Here, the cooking liquid is enhanced by fruit juice, cinnamon and cayenne pepper to enliven mild chicken breasts.

1 In large nonstick skillet combine ¾ cup apple juice, bouillon granules and garlic. Bring to boiling. Add chicken. Return to boiling. Reduce heat. Simmer, covered, for 7 minutes.

2 Add apple and cherries. Cover and simmer for 4 to 5 minutes more or until chicken is tender and no longer pink.

3 Use slotted spoon to remove chicken and fruit from liquid. Place on serving platter. Keep warm. Reserve liquid in skillet.

4 In small bowl stir together ⅓ cup apple juice, cornstarch, cinnamon and cayenne pepper. Stir into liquid in skillet. Cook and stir until boiling and thickened slightly. Spoon over chicken and fruit.

Make it a meal

Add these delicious side dishes to each serving to create a full meal (total additional calories: 365 per serving)

- Fennel and Quinoa Oven Pilaf (page 194)
- 1 cup steamed broccoli florets
- Grape juice spritzer (½ cup grape juice mixed with ½ cup sparkling water)

NUTRITION FACTS PER SERVING Calories: 240; Calories from Fat: 30; **Total Fat:** 3g; **Saturated Fat:** 0.5g; **Trans Fat:** 0g; **Cholesterol:** 75mg; **Sodium:** 200mg; **Total Carbohydrate:** 28g; **Dietary Fiber:** 5g; **Sugars:** 19g; **Protein:** 25g

Oven-Fried Chicken Cutlets

5 cups **Kellogg's®
Special K®** cereal
(crushed to 1²/₃ cups)

1 teaspoon poultry
seasoning

1 teaspoon dried
parsley leaves

¼ teaspoon garlic salt

¼ teaspoon paprika

¼ teaspoon pepper

²/₃ cup low-fat buttermilk

¹/₃ cup all-purpose flour

1 pound thin-sliced,
boneless, skinless chicken
breast cutlets

Olive oil cooking spray

¼ cup fat-free
plain yogurt

2 tablespoons spicy
brown mustard

Just as satisfying as deep-fried chicken, but with much less fat, this recipe is great for a family dinner. The cutlets are also delicious as sandwiches on toasted whole-wheat buns.

1 Preheat oven to 450°F.

2 Meanwhile, in shallow dish combine **Special K** cereal, poultry seasoning, parsley, garlic salt, paprika and pepper. Set aside.

3 Pour buttermilk into another shallow dish. Spread flour in even layer on sheet of wax paper.

4 Cut chicken into 6 serving-size pieces, if necessary. Lightly coat chicken with flour. Dip into buttermilk, coating both sides. Generously coat both sides with cereal mixture, lightly pressing crumbs into chicken. Place in single layer on baking sheet lined with foil and coated with cooking spray. Lightly coat tops of chicken pieces with additional cooking spray.

5 Bake chicken, uncovered, in preheated oven about 10 minutes or until lightly browned. Carefully turn chicken. Bake for 7 to 12 minutes more or until chicken is no longer pink.

6 Meanwhile, in small bowl stir together yogurt and mustard. Serve chicken with mustard mixture.

NUTRITION FACTS PER SERVING Calories: 240; **Calories from Fat:** 25; **Total Fat:** 3g; **Saturated Fat:** 1g; **Trans Fat:** 0g; **Cholesterol:** 50mg; **Sodium:** 400mg; **Total Carbohydrate:** 26g; **Dietary Fiber:** 1g; **Sugars:** 6g; **Protein:** 24g

Spicy Asian Chicken Stir-Fry

12 ounces medium rice noodles

Cooking spray

3 cups broccoli florets

3 cups red bell pepper strips

3 cups fresh snow peas

2 tablespoons vegetable oil

1½ pounds boneless, skinless chicken breasts, cut into bite-size pieces

1½ cups shredded carrots

1 cup plus 2 tablespoons bottled Thai-style peanut sauce

2 tablespoons reduced-sodium soy sauce

¾ teaspoon ground red pepper (optional)

4 tablespoons lightly salted dry-roasted peanuts, chopped

Featuring a wealth of vegetables, a sensible portion of noodles, just the right amount of lean protein, and a low-fat sauce, this recipe is a perfect, healthy one-dish meal.

1 Cook noodles according to package directions. Drain. Rinse with cold water. Drain well. Set aside.

2 In nonstick wok or large nonstick skillet coated with cooking spray, stir-fry broccoli and bell pepper over medium-high heat for 2 minutes. Stir in snow peas. Stir-fry for 1 minute longer. Remove vegetables from wok. Set aside.

3 Add oil to same wok. Add chicken. Stir-fry over medium-high heat for 2 to 3 minutes or until chicken is no longer pink. Reduce heat to medium. Return vegetables to wok. Stir in carrot, peanut sauce, soy sauce and ground red pepper (if desired). Add noodles. Toss until combined and heated through. Transfer to serving platter or individual plates. Sprinkle with peanuts.

Here's to your health

Some people steer clear of Asian-style dishes because they tend to be higher in sodium than those of other cuisines. If you're watching your own sodium intake, you can still make a delicious version of this recipe by replacing the soy sauce with lemon juice; and the Thai-style peanut sauce with 1 cup canned reduced-sodium chicken broth and 2 tablespoons unsalted peanut butter. Be sure to include the ground red pepper for its spicy zing.

NUTRITION FACTS PER SERVING Calories: 580; **Calories from Fat:** 140; **Total Fat:** 15g; **Saturated Fat:** 3g; **Trans Fat:** 0g; **Cholesterol:** 85mg; **Sodium:** 1090mg; **Total Carbohydrate:** 69g; **Dietary Fiber:** 6g; **Sugars:** 6g; **Protein:** 43g

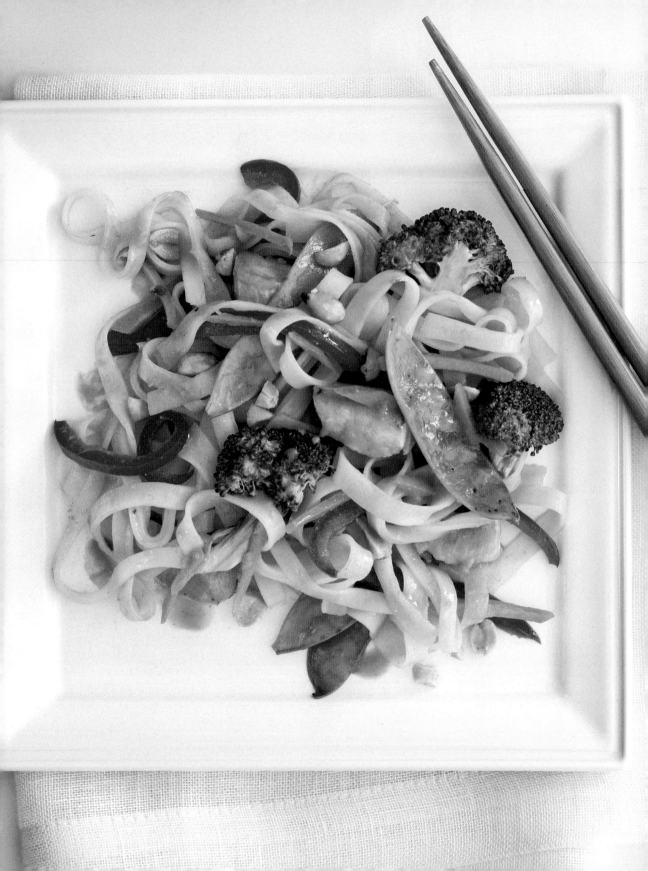

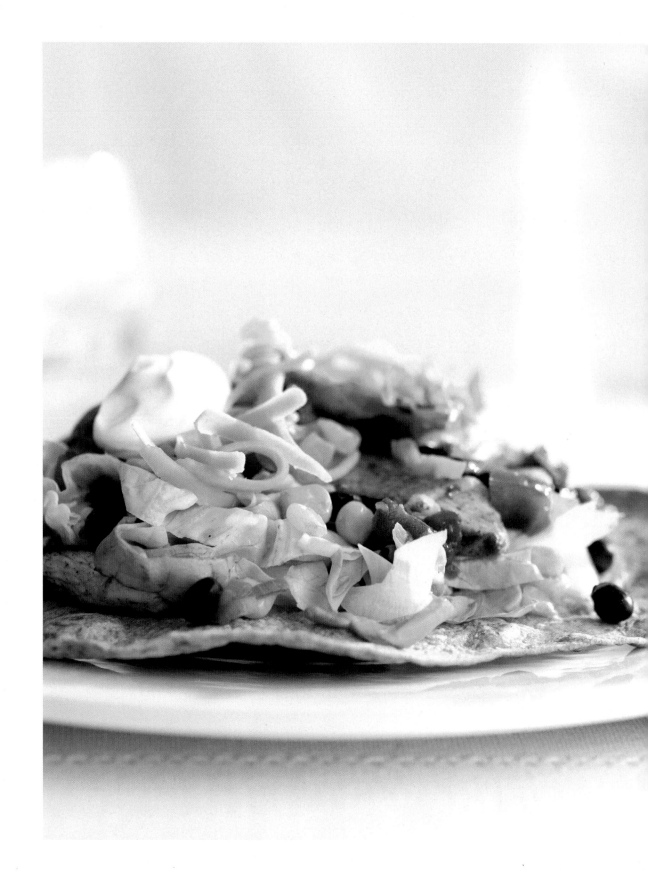

Roasted Corn AND Chicken Tostada

SERVES 4

Four 7-inch whole-wheat or flour tortillas

Cooking spray

1⅓ cups frozen whole-kernel corn

4 teaspoons vegetable oil

1 pound boneless, skinless chicken breasts, cut into bite-size pieces

2 teaspoons chili powder

1 teaspoon ground cumin

1 cup tomato salsa

1 cup canned black beans, rinsed and drained

4 cups shredded lettuce

½ cup shredded reduced-fat cheddar cheese

¼ cup nonfat sour cream

Here is a creative take on a popular Mexican dish, featuring a crisp, baked whole-wheat tortilla piled with a meaty salad and topped with low-fat cheese and sour cream.

1 Preheat oven to 400°F. Lightly coat both sides of tortillas with cooking spray. Place on baking sheet. Bake in preheated oven about 10 minutes or until tortillas are crisp.

2 Meanwhile, in large nonstick skillet coated with cooking spray, cook corn over medium-high heat, stirring frequently, for 1 to 3 minutes or until beginning to brown. Remove from skillet. Set aside.

3 In same skillet heat oil. Add chicken, chili powder and cumin. Cook and stir over medium-high heat for 2 to 3 minutes or until chicken is no longer pink. Stir in salsa, beans and corn. Heat through.

4 Place tortillas on serving plates. Top with lettuce, chicken mixture, cheese and sour cream. Serve immediately.

Make it a meal

Add these delicious side dishes to each serving to create a full meal (total additional calories: 270 per serving)

- 6 ounces low-fat lemon yogurt topped with ⅓ cup raspberries or blueberries
- 1 tablespoon reduced-fat, nondairy whipped topping
- ½ cup orange juice mixed with ½ to 1 cup sparkling water

NUTRITION FACTS PER SERVING Calories: 450; **Calories from Fat:** 130; **Total Fat:** 14g; **Saturated Fat:** 4g; **Trans Fat:** 0g; **Cholesterol:** 50mg; **Sodium:** 1540mg; **Total Carbohydrate:** 50g; **Dietary Fiber:** 10g; **Sugars:** 9g; **Protein:** 35g

Easy Chicken Potpies

1 medium leek

1 medium red potato (about 4 ounces)

⅓ cup finely chopped celery

⅓ cup finely chopped carrot

1 clove garlic, minced

1¼ cups reduced-sodium chicken broth

½ cup frozen cut green beans or frozen peas

¾ cup fat-free milk

3 tablespoons all-purpose flour

¼ teaspoon dried marjoram leaves

¼ teaspoon dried thyme leaves

¼ teaspoon salt

¼ teaspoon pepper

1½ cups chopped, rotisserie-roasted chicken breast (about 6 ounces)

1 package (7½ ounces; 10 count) refrigerated flaky-layers biscuit dough

When you need comfort food, but still want a healthy meal option, these vegetable-packed pies fit the bill. Purchased biscuit dough and rotisserie chicken make preparation easy.

1 Preheat oven to 400°F.

2 Trim and discard root ends from leek. Remove any tough outer leaves and most of the green portion of leek. Halve leek lengthwise and rinse layers thoroughly under cold running water. Cut leek into ¼-inch-thick slices.

3 Scrub potato. Cut into ½-inch pieces (you should have about 1 cup). In medium saucepan combine leek, potato, celery, carrot and garlic. Stir in broth and green beans. Bring to boiling. Reduce heat. Simmer, covered, about 15 minutes or until vegetables are tender.

4 In small bowl stir together milk, flour, marjoram, thyme, salt and pepper. Stir milk mixture and chicken into mixture in saucepan. Cook, stirring frequently, until mixture boils and thickens. Remove from heat. Cover to keep warm.

5 Cut each biscuit into fourths. Spoon chicken mixture into four 10- to 12-ounce ramekins or custard cups. Divide biscuit pieces among ramekins covering chicken mixture.

6 Place ramekins on baking sheet. Bake, uncovered, in preheated oven for 10 to 15 minutes or until tops are golden brown. Cool slightly before serving.

NUTRITION FACTS PER SERVING Calories: 320; Calories from Fat: 50; Total Fat: 6g; Saturated Fat: 1g; Trans Fat: 1g; Cholesterol: 45mg; Sodium: 700mg; Total Carbohydrate: 42g; Dietary Fiber: 3g; Sugars: 8g; Protein: 25g

Golden Crisp Chicken Salad

1 pound boneless, skinless chicken breast halves

1 egg white, slightly beaten

1 tablespoon water

½ teaspoon pepper seasoning salt

3 cups **Kellogg's®** **Special K®** Red Berries cereal (crushed to 1½ cups)

Cooking spray

1 package (10 ounces) prepared torn romaine lettuce

¼ cup fat-free raspberry vinaigrette

1 pear, cubed

¼ cup toasted pine nuts or slivered almonds (optional)

The oven-baked chicken strips that top this refreshing salad are crisp and succulent, with just a fraction of the fat and calories of their deep-fried cousins.

1 Preheat oven to 325°F.

2 Cut chicken lengthwise into 1-inch strips. In shallow bowl stir together egg white and water. Spread crushed **Special K** Red Berries cereal and pepper seasoning salt on plate. Dip chicken strips in egg whites, coating both sides. Generously coat both sides with cereal mixture, lightly pressing crumbs into chicken. Place in single layer on baking sheet lined with foil and coated with cooking spray. Sprinkle any remaining crumbs over chicken. Spray chicken pieces lightly with cooking spray.

3 Bake in preheated oven about 20 minutes or until chicken is tender and no longer pink. Do not cover pan or turn chicken while baking.

4 Toss romaine with vinaigrette and portion onto serving plates. Place hot chicken strips over romaine and sprinkle with pear and nuts (if desired). Serve immediately.

NUTRITION FACTS PER SERVING Calories: 320; Calories from Fat: 70; **Total Fat:** 7g; **Saturated Fat:** 1g; **Trans Fat:** 0g; **Cholesterol:** 65mg; **Sodium:** 330mg; **Total Carbohydrate:** 35g; **Dietary Fiber:** 5g; **Sugars:** 15g; **Protein:** 31g

Jamaican Chicken Breast
WITH Mashed Sweet Potatoes

4 small sweet potatoes
(about 6 ounces each)

4 small boneless, skinless
chicken breast halves
(about 5 ounces each)

1 teaspoon vegetable oil

4 teaspoons Caribbean
jerk seasoning

Cooking spray

2 cups canned
black beans, rinsed
and drained

2 cups chopped tomato

1 cup reduced-sodium
chicken broth

4 tablespoons sliced
green onions

2 teaspoons butter
or margarine

Caribbean-style jerk seasonings deliver bold flavor to this colorful chicken dish, which is accented by mashed sweet potatoes and a warm black bean salsa.

1 Scrub potatoes. Trim ends. Prick skin in several places with fork. Place in shallow microwave-safe dish. Loosely cover with plastic wrap and micro-cook at high for 12 to 16 minutes or until very tender, turning dish every 2 minutes. Let potatoes stand until cool enough to handle.

2 Meanwhile, brush chicken breasts on both sides with oil. Rub jerk seasoning on both sides.

3 In small nonstick skillet coated with cooking spray cook chicken over medium-low heat about 6 minutes or until lightly browned, turning once. Add beans, tomato and broth to skillet. Bring to boiling. Reduce heat. Simmer, covered, about 5 minutes or until chicken is no longer pink. Stir onions into bean mixture.

4 Meanwhile, use spoon to scoop pulp from potatoes. Slightly mash pulp. Stir in butter. Return to microwave-safe dish. Micro-cook, loosely covered, about 1 minute or until heated through. Spoon onto serving plates. Top with chicken and vegetables. Serve immediately.

NUTRITION FACTS PER SERVING Calories: 410; Calories from Fat: 45; **Total Fat:** 5g; **Saturated Fat:** 2g; **Trans Fat:** 0g; **Cholesterol:** 90mg; **Sodium:** 1140mg; **Total Carbohydrate:** 51g; **Dietary Fiber:** 13g; **Sugars:** 13g; **Protein:** 42g

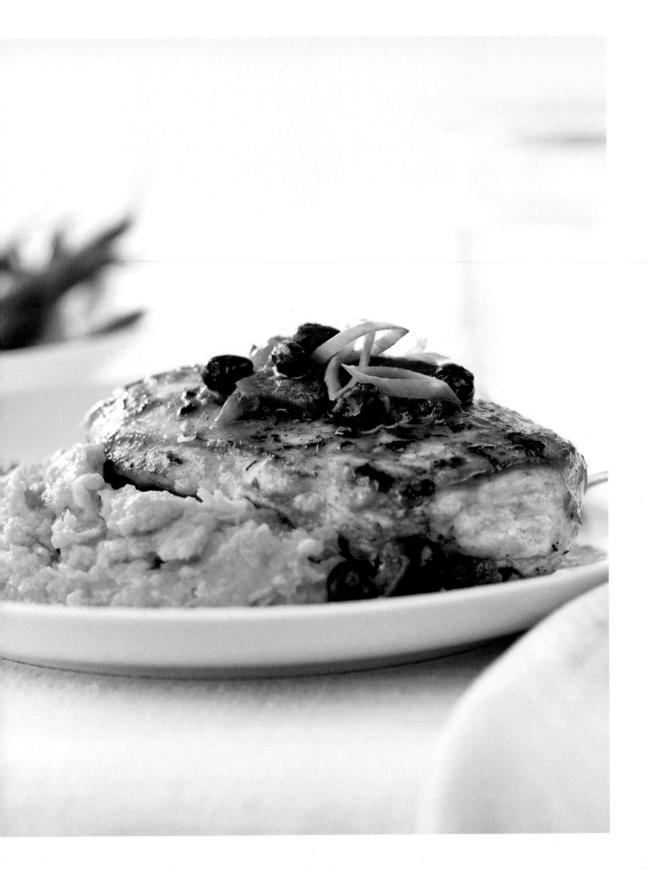

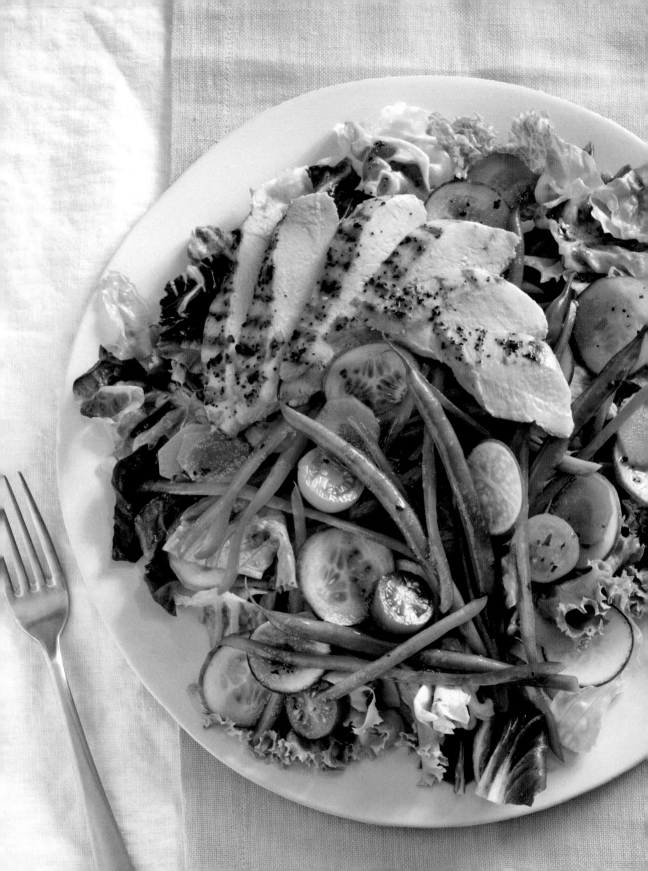

Grilled Chicken Salad

SERVES 4

4 ounces fresh green beans, trimmed

4 medium boneless, skinless chicken breast halves (about 6 ounces each)

4 teaspoons olive oil

1 teaspoon garlic pepper seasoning blend

8 cups torn mixed greens

2 medium carrots, shaved into thin slices

1 medium red bell pepper, seeded and cut into slivers

1 cup sliced cucumber

4 radishes, sliced

2 cups halved yellow or red grape tomatoes or cherry tomatoes

¾ cup reduced-fat balsamic vinaigrette

Here, seasoned grilled chicken tops a plateful of fresh vegetables and greens, which are drizzled with reduced-fat dressing. Substitute your favorite vegetables as you like.

1 Preheat grill or broiler.

2 In large saucepan plunge green beans into boiling water for 10 minutes or until crisp-tender. Drain. Cool.

3 Brush chicken on both sides with olive oil. Sprinkle with garlic pepper seasoning. Grill chicken directly over medium heat for 12 to 15 minutes or until tender and no longer pink, turning once. Alternatively, place on rack of broiler pan 4 to 5 inches from heat for 12 to 15 minutes, turning once. Cut chicken into slices.

4 Place greens on serving plates. Arrange green beans, carrots, bell pepper, cucumber and radishes on top. Sprinkle with tomatoes. Top with chicken. Serve with balsamic vinaigrette.

Make it a meal

Add these delicious side dishes to each serving to create a full meal (total additional calories: 450 per serving)

- 1 whole-wheat dinner roll with 2 teaspoons butter
- 1 cup low-fat chocolate sorbet with ½ cup red raspberries
- 2 tablespoons reduced-fat nondairy whipped topping

NUTRITION FACTS PER SERVING Calories: 330; Calories from Fat: 80; **Total Fat:** 9g; **Saturated Fat:** 1.5g; **Trans Fat:** 0g; **Cholesterol:** 100mg; **Sodium:** 1050mg; **Total Carbohydrate:** 25g; **Dietary Fiber:** 6g; **Sugars:** 11g; **Protein:** 43g

Italian-Style Parmesan Chicken

SERVES 4

1 cup **Kellogg's®
Special K®** cereal

1 tablespoon
all-purpose flour

2 tablespoons grated
Parmesan cheese

2 teaspoons
Italian seasoning

⅓ cup reduced-calorie
Italian salad dressing

4 boneless, skinless
chicken breast halves
(about 1 pound total)

Cooking spray

Here, a simple quartet of ingredients—Italian seasoning blend, **Special K** cereal, Parmesan cheese and Italian dressing—make a dish reminiscent of chicken Parmigiana.

1 Preheat oven to 350°F.

2 In food processor work bowl or blender container, combine **Special K** cereal, flour, Parmesan cheese and Italian seasoning until cereal is in fine crumbs. Place mixture in shallow pan. Set aside.

3 Pour salad dressing into another shallow pan. Dip chicken in salad dressing, coating both sides. Generously coat both sides with cereal mixture, lightly pressing crumbs into chicken. Place in single layer in shallow baking pan coated with cooking spray.

4 Bake in preheated oven about 30 minutes or until tender and no longer pink. Do not cover or turn chicken while baking.

NUTRITION FACTS PER SERVING Calories: 220; Calories from Fat: 80; **Total Fat:** 9g; **Saturated Fat:** 2.5g; **Trans Fat:** 0g; **Cholesterol:** 75mg; **Sodium:** 350mg; **Total Carbohydrate:** 7g; **Dietary Fiber:** 0g; **Sugars:** 2g; **Protein:** 26g

Curried Chicken Salad

3 cups chopped, cooked chicken breast

2 cups seedless red grapes, halved, and/or fresh blueberries

2 cups sliced celery

⅓ cup sliced green onions

½ cup nonfat plain yogurt

¼ cup reduced-fat mayonnaise

2 teaspoons reduced-sodium soy sauce

2 teaspoons curry powder

⅛ teaspoon garlic powder

6 lettuce leaves

1½ cups **Kellogg's® Special K®** Red Berries cereal

You can make this easy and delicious salad with leftover chicken or with cooked rotisserie chicken breast from the market. Remove all skin and fat from the meat before using.

1 In large bowl toss together chicken, grapes, celery and onions.

2 In small bowl stir together yogurt, mayonnaise, soy sauce, curry powder and garlic powder. Pour over chicken mixture. Toss to coat. Cover and refrigerate at least 2 hours.

3 Stir chicken mixture. Divide among 6 lettuce-lined salad plates. Top with cereal and serve immediately.

Make it your own

Curry spices and fresh, sweet fruit pair up delightfully in main-dish salads. Try these tasty substitutions for the grapes or blueberries in this recipe:

Autumn Curried Chicken Salad Use 2 cups diced fresh apple, pear or a mixture of the two

Tropical Curried Chicken Salad Use 2 cups mixed fresh tropical fruit such as pineapple, mango, papaya or banana

Curried Chicken Salad with Dried Fruit Use 1 cup mixed dried fruit such as seedless raisins or dried apricots, peaches, apples or pears

NUTRITION FACTS PER SERVING Calories: 240; **Calories from Fat:** 50; **Total Fat:** 6g; **Saturated Fat:** 1.5g; **Trans Fat:** 0g; **Cholesterol:** 65mg; **Sodium:** 270mg; **Total Carbohydrate:** 21g; **Dietary Fiber:** 2g; **Sugars:** 13g; **Protein:** 25g

Mediterranean Turkey Sandwiches

SERVES 4

½ cup roasted garlic hummus or plain hummus

8 slices whole-grain bread

½ teaspoon pepper

4 lettuce leaves

¾ pound thinly sliced roasted turkey breast

1 cup thinly sliced cucumber

1 cup thinly sliced red bell pepper strips

These hearty turkey sandwiches gain extra nutrition with their stuffing of thinly sliced crisp vegetables. The usual sandwich spread is replaced by nutrient-packed hummus.

1 Spread the hummus on one side of each bread slice. Lightly sprinkle hummus with pepper.

2 Evenly distribute lettuce leaves, sliced turkey, cucumber and bell pepper on top of 4 slices. Top with remaining bread, hummus side down. Cut each sandwich in half and serve.

Make it a meal

Add these delicious side dishes to each serving to create a full meal (total additional calories: 360 per serving)

- A salad made of 3 or 4 slices yellow, orange or red tomatoes and 2 ounces sliced fresh mozzarella cheese

- Top tomatoes and cheese with 2 teaspoons balsamic vinegar and 2 teaspoons chopped fresh basil

- 1½ cups red grapes

NUTRITION FACTS PER SERVING Calories: 290; Calories from Fat: 60; **Total Fat:** 7g; **Saturated Fat:** 1g; **Trans Fat:** 0g; **Cholesterol:** 35mg; **Sodium:** 1200mg; **Total Carbohydrate:** 35g; **Dietary Fiber:** 6g; **Sugars:** 8g; **Protein:** 23g

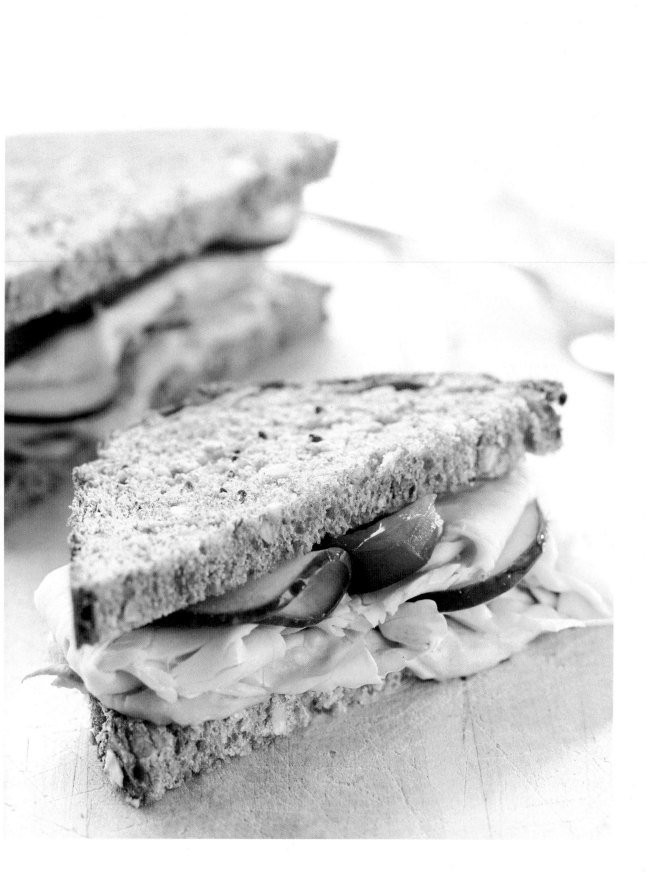

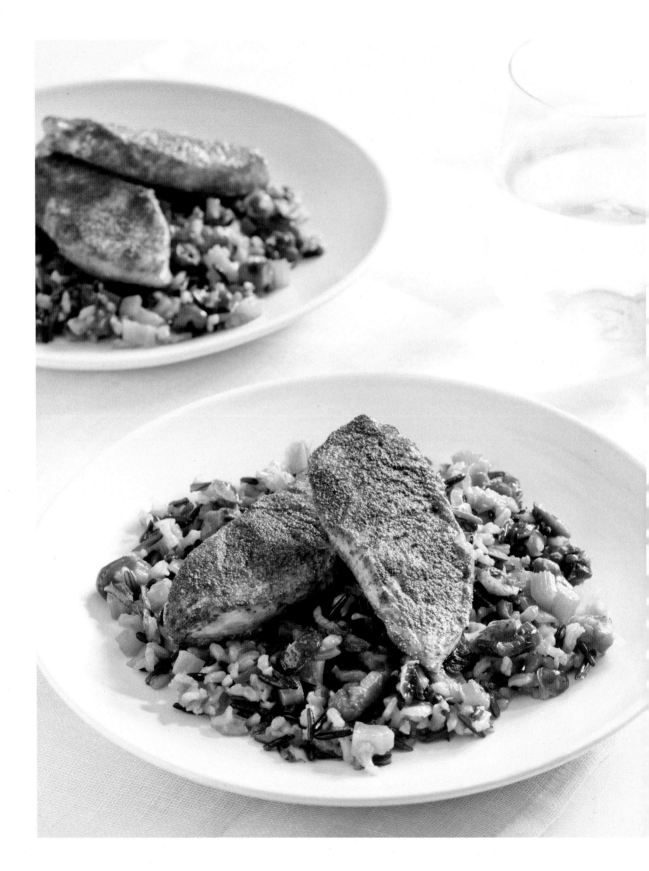

Spiced Turkey Cutlets WITH Cranberry–Wild Rice Pilaf

SERVES 4

Cooking spray

½ cup wild rice, rinsed and drained

½ cup long-grain brown rice

½ cup dried cranberries

¼ cup chopped walnuts, toasted

2 stalks celery, chopped (about 1 cup)

¼ cup chopped onion

2 teaspoons butter or margarine

1¼ cups reduced-sodium chicken broth

1 cup apple juice

¾ teaspoon ground cumin

½ teaspoon cinnamon

¼ teaspoon salt

⅛ teaspoon garlic powder

⅛ teaspoon cayenne pepper

One 12-ounce turkey breast tenderloin, cut into ¾-inch-thick pieces

Although this one-dish meal boasts flavors reminiscent of Thanksgiving—turkey, cinnamon, cranberries and walnuts—it makes a perfect main dish at any time of the year.

1 Preheat oven to 350°F.

2 Meanwhile, in 8 x 8 x 2-inch baking dish coated with cooking spray combine wild rice, brown rice, cranberries and walnuts. In medium saucepan cook celery and onion in butter over medium heat until tender. Add broth and apple juice. Bring to boiling. Pour over rice mixture. Tightly cover with foil. Bake in preheated oven for 50 minutes.

3 Meanwhile, in small bowl stir together cumin, cinnamon, salt, garlic powder and cayenne pepper. Rub on both sides of turkey pieces.

4 Uncover rice. Stir. Top with turkey pieces. Tightly cover again with foil. Bake in preheated oven for 15 minutes. Remove foil. Bake, uncovered, at 350°F for 5 minutes more or until most of liquid is absorbed and turkey is no longer pink.

5 To serve, spoon rice mixture onto individual serving plates, topping with turkey pieces.

NUTRITION FACTS PER SERVING Calories: 430; Calories from Fat: 110; Total Fat: 12g; Saturated Fat: 4g; Trans Fat: 0g; Cholesterol: 45mg; Sodium: 290mg; Total Carbohydrate: 57g; Dietary Fiber: 5g; Sugars: 19g; Protein: 29g

Orange-Glazed Stuffed Turkey Breast

3 tablespoons Dijon mustard or spicy brown mustard

2 tablespoons frozen orange juice concentrate, thawed

2½ cups fresh whole-wheat breadcrumbs

½ cup chopped pecans, toasted

⅓ cup finely chopped dried apricots or dried tart cherries

¼ cup chopped celery

¼ cup orange juice

2 teaspoons grated orange zest

½ teaspoon dried sage leaves

¼ teaspoon salt

1 clove garlic, minced

One 3- to 3½-pound boneless whole turkey breast

This delivers all the flavor of a holiday turkey, without all the fuss. If your market has only bone-in turkey breasts, ask the butcher to bone one for you, leaving the halves attached.

1 Preheat oven to 325°F.

2 In small bowl stir together mustard and orange juice concentrate. Cover and refrigerate until needed.

3 In small bowl stir together breadcrumbs, pecans, apricots, celery, orange juice, orange zest, sage, salt and garlic.

4 Place turkey breast, skin side down, on cutting board. Spoon breadcrumb mixture between breast halves. Roll turkey around stuffing. Securely tie with kitchen string.

5 Place turkey breast, skin side up, on rack in shallow roasting pan. Roast, uncovered, in preheated oven for 1¾ to 2¼ hours or until instant-read thermometer inserted into thickest part of breast registers 170°F and thermometer inserted into stuffing registers 165°F. Brush with mustard mixture during the last 30 minutes of roasting. Let stand for 10 minutes before carving. Serve warm.

NUTRITION FACTS PER SERVING Calories: 320; Calories from Fat: 130; Total Fat: 14g; Saturated Fat: 3g; Trans Fat: 0g; Cholesterol: 100mg; Sodium: 280mg; Total Carbohydrate: 11g; Dietary Fiber: 2g; Sugars: 5g; Protein: 35g

Turkey Meatloaf
WITH Barbecue Sauce

SERVES 8

Barbecue Sauce

½ cup ketchup

3 tablespoons honey

1 tablespoon
prepared mustard

2 tablespoons vinegar

Turkey Meatloaf

2 egg whites

2 cups **Kellogg's®
Special K®** cereal

2 tablespoons
chopped onion

1 teaspoon salt

¼ teaspoon pepper

1½ pounds lean
ground turkey

Lean ground turkey, **Special K** cereal, egg whites and a quick homemade barbecue sauce add up to one of the tastiest and healthiest versions of meatloaf you'll find.

1 Preheat oven to 350°F.

2 To make barbecue sauce, in small bowl stir together ketchup, honey, mustard and vinegar; stir to combine. Set aside.

3 In large bowl, beat egg whites until foamy. Add **Special K** cereal, onion, salt, pepper and ½ cup Barbecue Sauce; beat well. Add ground turkey; mix gently until combined. Shape turkey mixture into loaf on shallow baking pan lined with foil. Score top by making diagonal grooves with knife; fill grooves and brush top with remaining barbecue sauce.

4 Bake in preheated oven about 1 hour or until instant-read thermometer inserted into thickest part of loaf registers 160°F. Let stand for a few minutes. Slice to serve.

Make it a meal

Add these delicious side dishes to each serving to create a full meal (total additional calories: 324 per serving)

- Whipped Buttermilk Potatoes (page 203)
- 1 cup steamed green beans
- Red Velvet Cupcake (page 222)

NUTRITION FACTS PER SERVING Calories: 200; Calories from Fat: 70; **Total Fat:** 7g; **Saturated Fat:** 2g; **Trans Fat:** 0g; **Cholesterol:** 65mg; **Sodium:** 650mg; **Total Carbohydrate:** 17g; **Dietary Fiber:** less than 1g; **Sugars:** 9g; **Protein:** 18g

Turkey Meatballs WITH Spaghetti IN Spicy Tomato Sauce

SERVES 6

1 egg white

2 tablespoons water

2 teaspoons ancho chili powder or other pure chili powder

¼ teaspoon black pepper

¼ teaspoon salt

1 cup fresh whole-wheat breadcrumbs

1 cup finely chopped onion

1 jalapeño chili, seeded and finely chopped

1 pound lean ground turkey

8 ounces dried whole-wheat spaghetti

1 cup chopped carrot

2 cloves garlic, minced

1 teaspoon vegetable oil

1 can (28 ounces) fire-roasted crushed tomatoes or regular crushed tomatoes

2 tablespoons tomato paste

2 teaspoons dried oregano leaves

⅛ teaspoon cayenne pepper

Not your ordinary spaghetti and meatballs, this lean, juicy and flavorful version gets a subtle, satisfying kick from chili powder and a fresh jalapeño chili blended into the meatballs.

1 Preheat oven to 375°F.

2 For meatballs, in medium bowl whisk together egg white, water, ½ teaspoon of the chili powder, black pepper and salt. Stir in breadcrumbs, ¼ cup of the onion and jalapeño chili. Add ground turkey. Mix gently until combined.

3 Shape turkey mixture into eighteen 1½-inch meatballs. Place on 15 x 10 x 1-inch baking pan. Bake in preheated oven about 20 minutes or until no longer pink. Remove from oven and set aside.

4 Meanwhile, cook pasta according to package directions. Drain. Rinse with cold water. Drain well.

5 For sauce, in nonstick Dutch oven cook remaining onion, carrot and garlic in oil over medium heat until tender. Stir in remaining chili powder, tomatoes with their juices, tomato paste, oregano and cayenne pepper. Bring to boiling. Reduce heat. Simmer, uncovered, about 15 minutes or until thickened to a sauce consistency.

6 Stir meatballs into sauce and simmer briefly until meatballs have heated through. Add pasta. Toss gently together to coat pasta with sauce, taking care not to break meatballs. Using pasta servers, transfer to serving bowls.

NUTRITION FACTS PER SERVING Calories: 320; Calories from Fat: 60; Total Fat: 6g; Saturated Fat: 1.5g; Trans Fat: 0g; Cholesterol: 45mg; Sodium: 580mg; Total Carbohydrate: 47g; Dietary Fiber: 9g; Sugars: 11g; Protein: 24g

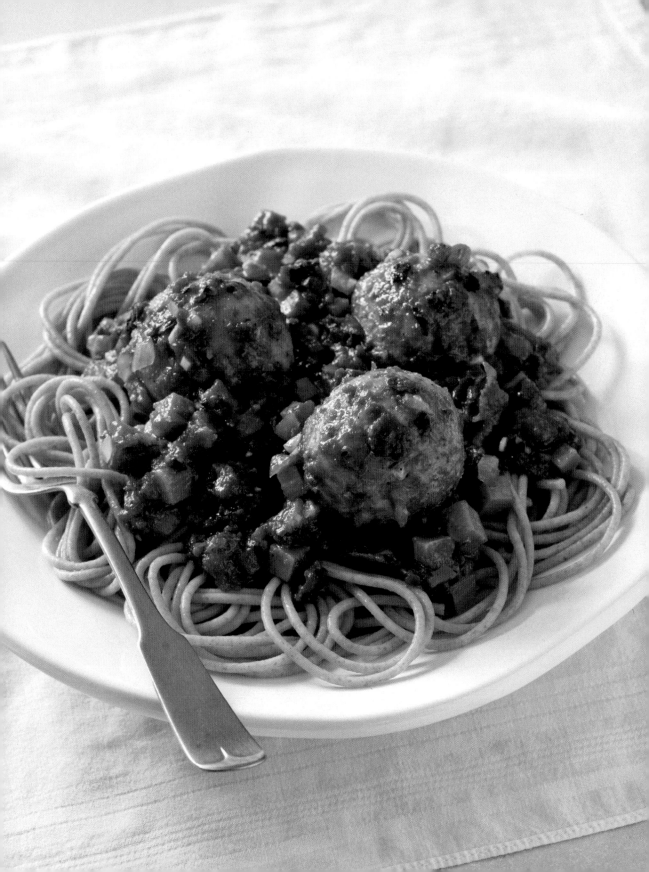

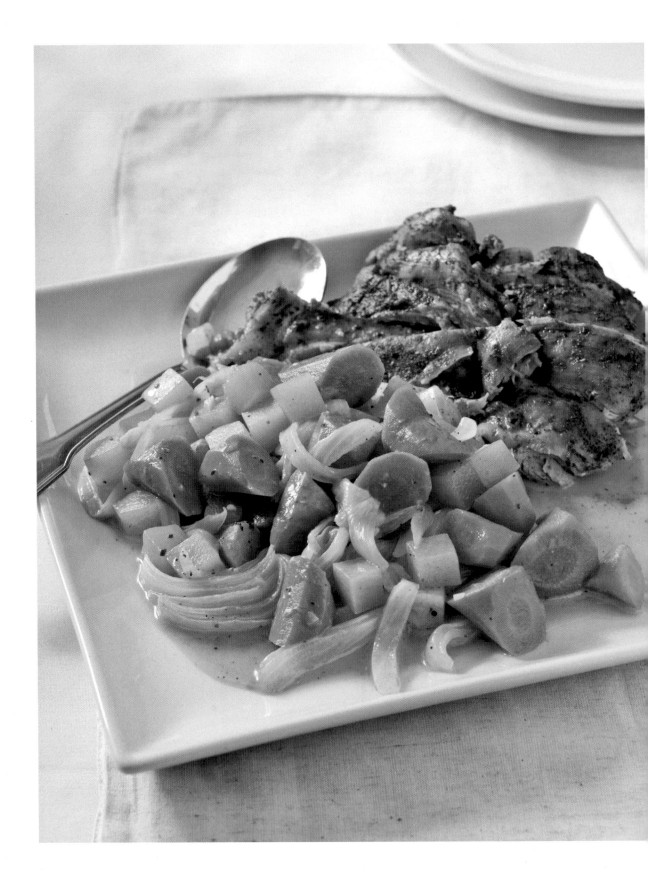

Braised Turkey Thighs
WITH Winter Root Vegetables

SERVES 4

1 teaspoon poultry
seasoning

¼ teaspoon salt

¼ teaspoon pepper

Two 1¼-pound turkey
thighs, skin and excess
fat removed

1 teaspoon vegetable oil

1 cup reduced-sodium
chicken broth

3 tablespoons apple juice

1 clove garlic, minced

5 medium carrots,
cut into 1-inch pieces
(about 2 cups)

2 medium turnips,
cut into ½-inch pieces
(about 2 cups)

1 medium onion, cut
into narrow wedges

⅛ teaspoon paprika

Long, slow cooking makes these turkey thighs extra tender. Removing the skin and any visible fat before cooking makes the flavorful dark meat a lean choice.

1 In small bowl combine poultry seasoning, salt and pepper. Rub on turkey thighs. In nonstick Dutch oven quickly brown turkey in oil over medium-high heat, turning frequently. Drain off any fat.

2 Add broth, apple juice and garlic to turkey thighs. Bring to boiling. Reduce heat. Simmer, covered, for 50 minutes. Add carrots, turnips and onion. Cover and simmer for 25 to 30 minutes more or until turkey and vegetables are tender. Transfer vegetables to serving platter. Cover to keep warm.

3 Remove turkey from Dutch oven to cutting board. Cut turkey meat from bones in large pieces. Add meat to vegetables on serving platter. Pour cooking liquid into measuring cup or gravy separator. Skim and discard any fat from liquid. Drizzle about ⅓ cup of the liquid over turkey and vegetables. Sprinkle turkey with paprika. Serve immediately.

NUTRITION FACTS PER SERVING Calories: 270; Calories from Fat: 80; **Total Fat:** 9g; **Saturated Fat:** 2.5g; **Trans Fat:** 0g; **Cholesterol:** 0mg; **Sodium:** 370mg; **Total Carbohydrate:** 18g; **Dietary Fiber:** 5g; **Sugars:** 12g; **Protein:** 42g

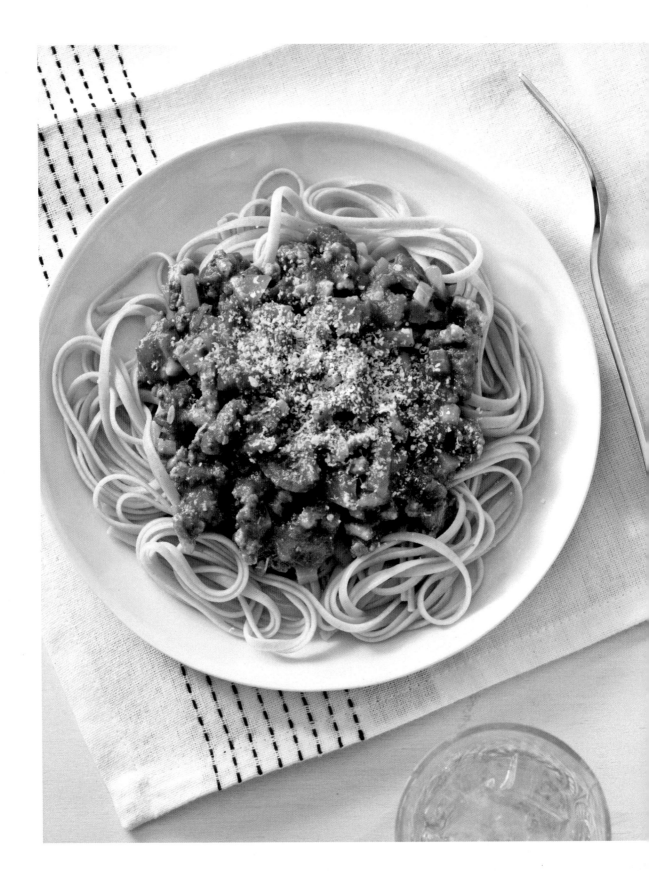

Meat Main Dishes

Sichuan Orange Beef-and-Broccoli Stir-Fry 158

Seared Steak Salad 161

Lean Beef Meatloaf 162

Beef Stew with Mushrooms 163

Open-Face Roast Beef Sandwiches 164

Pasta with Bolognese Sauce 167

Sautéed Veal with Balsamic Sauce 168

Pork Chops with Pomegranate Glaze 169

Moroccan Lamb and Chickpea Stew 170

Pork Posole 173

Asian Pork, Noodle and Bok Choy Stir-Fry 174

Pork Stew with Root Vegetables and Dried Fruits 175

Sichuan Orange Beef-
and-Broccoli Stir-Fry

SERVES 4

⅓ cup orange juice

¼ cup reduced-sodium
soy sauce

1 tablespoon hoisin sauce

2 teaspoons cornstarch

2 teaspoons grated
fresh ginger

1 teaspoon grated
orange zest

¾ teaspoon crushed
red pepper

½ teaspoon sugar

2 cloves garlic, minced

2 teaspoons vegetable oil

½ large onion,
cut into thin slivers
(about 1½ cups)

1 cup sliced carrot

3 cups broccoli florets

8 ounces beef sirloin
steak, trimmed and cut
into ⅛-inch-thick slices

1 cup fresh sugar
snap peas

2 cups hot cooked
brown rice

Bold flavors make this easy, low-fat, Chinese-style stir-fry
intensely satisfying. Orange juice contributes tangy sweetness,
while crushed red pepper adds spicy fire.

1 In small bowl stir together orange juice, soy sauce, hoisin sauce,
cornstarch, ginger, orange zest, crushed red pepper, sugar and garlic.
Cover with plastic wrap and set aside.

2 Heat 1 teaspoon of the oil in nonstick wok or large nonstick skillet
over high heat. Add onion. Stir-fry for 2 minutes. Add carrot. Stir-fry
for 2 minutes more. Add broccoli. Stir-fry for 2 to 3 minutes or until
vegetables are crisp-tender. Remove from wok.

3 Add remaining oil to wok. Stir-fry beef for 2 to 3 minutes or until
desired doneness. Stir orange juice mixture. Add to wok. Cook, stirring
constantly, until mixture boils. Stir in vegetable mixture and pea
pods. Heat through. Serve over rice.

Make it your own

This luscious stir-fry recipe is easy to vary to your
personal taste. In place of any of the vegetables listed,
try other favorites such as cauliflower florets, bite-sized
pieces of asparagus, green beans or whole baby spinach
leaves (add these towards the very end of stirring).
For the beef, substitute thinly sliced lean pork or lamb.
Or, make a vegetarian version using firm tofu, drained
well and cut into ½-inch cubes.

NUTRITION FACTS PER SERVING Calories: 300; Calories from Fat: 50; **Total Fat:** 6g; **Saturated Fat:** 1.5g; **Trans Fat:** 0g;
Cholesterol: 20mg; **Sodium:** 670mg; **Total Carbohydrate:** 45g; **Dietary Fiber:** 7g; **Sugars:** 10g; **Protein:** 18g

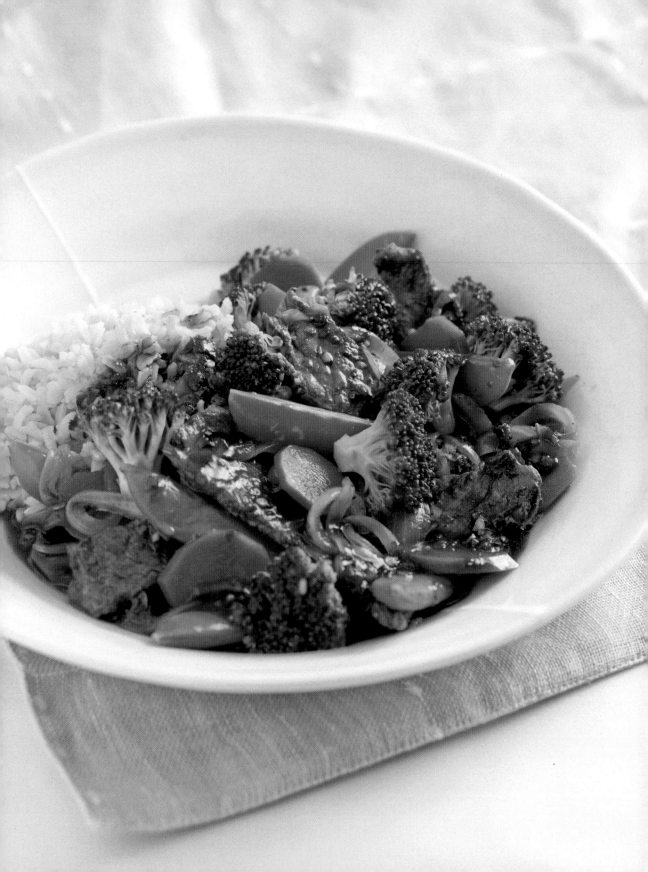

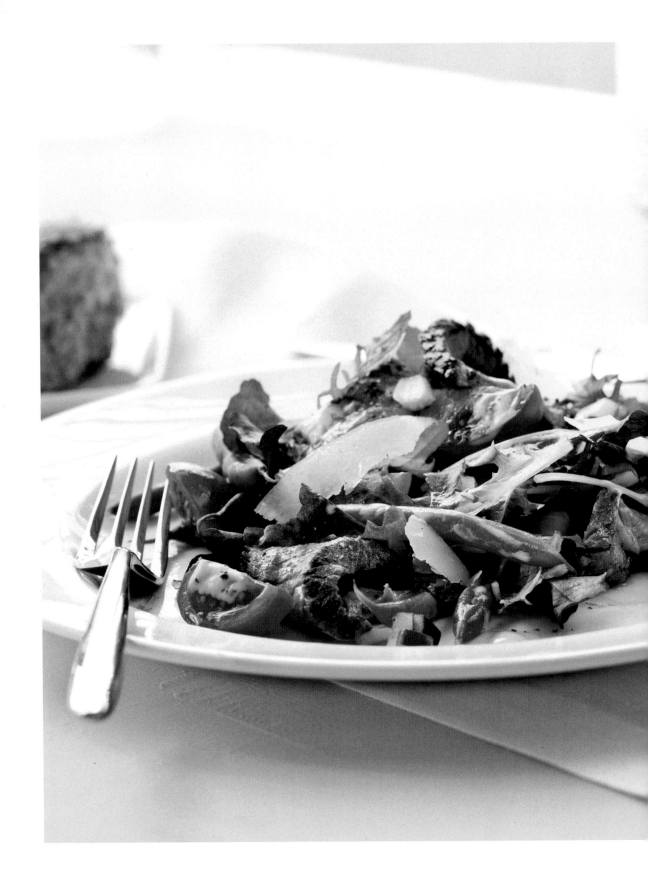

Seared Steak Salad

SERVES 4

4 ounces fresh green beans, trimmed

8 cups torn mixed greens

2 cups quartered grape tomatoes or cherry tomatoes

¾ cup bottled fat-free creamy Caesar salad dressing

2 teaspoons ground cumin

½ teaspoon salt

½ teaspoon pepper

1 pound boneless sirloin steak, cut 1 inch thick, trimmed

Olive oil cooking spray

2 teaspoons lemon juice

4 tablespoons chopped red onion

1 ounce shaved Parmesan cheese

In this recipe, slices of spice-rubbed steak are draped over fresh vegetables, then garnished with shavings of Parmesan cheese for a robust main-dish salad low in calories and fat.

1 In large saucepan plunge green beans into boiling water for 10 minutes or until crisp-tender. Drain. Rinse under cold running water until cool. Drain again.

2 In medium bowl combine greens, tomatoes and salad dressing. Add green beans. Toss until combined. Arrange on serving plates.

3 In small bowl stir together cumin, salt and pepper. Rub on both sides of steak. In nonstick skillet coated with cooking spray, cook steak over medium heat for 9 to 12 minutes, turning once, or until desired doneness. Remove from skillet. With sharp knife cut steak across grain into thin slices. Arrange slices on top of green salads.

4 Sprinkle lemon juice over steak slices. Top with onion and shaved Parmesan. Serve immediately.

Make it a meal

Add these delicious side dishes to each serving to create a full meal (total additional calories: 396 per serving)

- One 2½-inch whole-wheat dinner roll

- 1 teaspoon butter

- 1 medium nectarine (about 1 cup sliced) or other fresh fruit, topped with 6 ounces nonfat vanilla yogurt and nutmeg

- Unsweetened iced tea with lemon wedge

NUTRITION FACTS PER SERVING Calories: 260; **Calories from Fat:** 80; **Total Fat:** 9g; **Saturated Fat:** 3g; **Trans Fat:** 0g; **Cholesterol:** 50mg; **Sodium:** 960mg; **Total Carbohydrate:** 18g; **Dietary Fiber:** 4g; **Sugars:** 11g; **Protein:** 28g

Lean Beef Meatloaf

3 cups **Kellogg's®
Special K®** cereal

1½ pounds lean
ground beef

1 egg, slightly beaten

½ cup finely
chopped onion

½ cup finely sliced celery

½ cup stewed tomatoes

½ cup fat-free milk

1½ teaspoons salt

⅛ teaspoon pepper

This meatloaf recipe makes it possible to enjoy good, old-fashioned, home-style comfort food without the guilt. Save leftovers for sandwiches on multigrain bread.

1 Preheat oven to 375°F.

2 In medium mixing bowl, combine **Special K** cereal, beef, egg, onion, celery, tomatoes, milk, salt and pepper. Mix gently until combined. Pack lightly in ungreased 9 x 5 x 3-inch loaf pan.

3 Bake in preheated oven about 1 hour or until an instant-read thermometer inserted into the thickest part of the loaf registers 160°F. Let stand 5 minutes before turning out onto heated platter. Slice and serve immediately.

Make it a meal

Add these delicious side dishes to each serving to create a full meal (total additional calories: 364 per serving)

- Roasted Cauliflower and Tomatoes (page 196)
- 1 cup cooked enriched dry egg noodles tossed with 1 teaspoon unsalted butter
- 1 cup mixed fresh fruit salad garnished with 1 tablespoon chopped walnuts

NUTRITION FACTS PER SERVING Calories: 210; Calories from Fat: 80; **Total Fat:** 8g; **Saturated Fat:** 3.5g; **Trans Fat:** 0g; **Cholesterol:** 60mg; **Sodium:** 620mg; **Total Carbohydrate:** 11g; **Dietary Fiber:** less than 1g; **Sugars:** 3g; **Protein:** 21g

Beef Stew with Mushrooms

SERVES 6

1½ pounds boneless beef top round steak, cut ¾ inch thick

2 teaspoons vegetable oil

2 cloves garlic, minced

4½ cups reduced-sodium beef broth

2 tablespoons balsamic vinegar

½ teaspoon dried marjoram leaves

½ teaspoon dried thyme leaves

½ teaspoon salt

¼ teaspoon pepper

4 medium red potatoes, cut into 1-inch pieces (about 4 cups)

3 cups quartered fresh mushrooms (about 8 ounces)

1½ cups baby carrots

1½ cups frozen pearl onions

¼ cup all-purpose flour

2 tablespoons tomato paste

Chopped fresh parsley (optional)

Long, slow cooking renders a lean cut of beef meltingly tender. Here, it's combined with a variety of fresh vegetables to create a healthy stew that is perfect for a chilly evening.

1 Cut beef into ¾- to 1-inch pieces. In nonstick Dutch oven quickly brown half of beef in oil over medium-high heat. Remove beef from Dutch oven. Add remaining beef and garlic to Dutch oven. Cook, stirring frequently, until browned. Return all beef to Dutch oven.

2 Stir in 4 cups of the broth, vinegar, marjoram, thyme, salt and pepper. Bring to boiling. Reduce heat. Simmer, covered, for 30 minutes. Stir in potatoes, mushrooms, carrots and onions. Return to boiling. Reduce heat. Simmer, covered, for 30 to 40 minutes or until beef and vegetables are tender.

3 In small bowl stir together remaining broth, flour and tomato paste. Stir into beef mixture. Cook, uncovered, over medium-high heat until mixture boils and thickens slightly, stirring frequently. Boil for 1 minute.

4 Ladle into serving bowls. Sprinkle with parsley (if desired).

NUTRITION FACTS PER SERVING Calories: 290; Calories from Fat: 60; Total Fat: 6g; Saturated Fat: 2g; Trans Fat: 0g; Cholesterol: 50mg; Sodium: 380mg; Total Carbohydrate: 32g; Dietary Fiber: 3g; Sugars: 7g; Protein: 32g

Open-Face Roast Beef Sandwiches

8 teaspoons nonfat plain yogurt or nonfat sour cream

4 teaspoons reduced-fat mayonnaise

4 teaspoons prepared horseradish

4 slices multigrain bread, toasted

2 cups mixed baby spring greens

12 ounces thinly sliced lean roast beef

4 tablespoons crumbled blue cheese

A satisfying roast beef sandwich takes a healthy turn by using lean meat, mixing nonfat yogurt or sour cream with reduced-fat mayonnaise and using only one slice of bread.

1 In small mixing bowl stir together yogurt, mayonnaise and horseradish. Spread on toast.

2 Top each slice of toast with greens, roast beef and blue cheese.

Make it a meal

Add these delicious side dishes to each serving to create a full meal (total additional calories: 402 per serving)

- Tomato, black bean and corn salad with 1 tablespoon Italian dressing
- 24 **Special K** crackers
- 1 large banana

NUTRITION FACTS PER SERVING Calories: 230; Calories from Fat: 80; Total Fat: 9g; Saturated Fat: 3.5g; Trans Fat: 0g; Cholesterol: 60mg; Sodium: 790mg; Total Carbohydrate: 15g; Dietary Fiber: 3g; Sugars: 3g; Protein: 24g

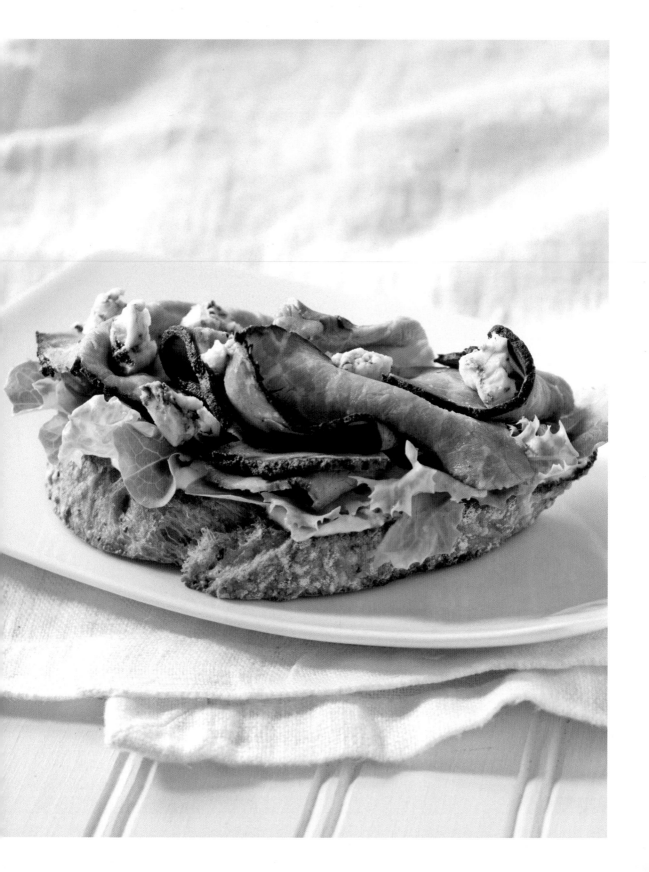

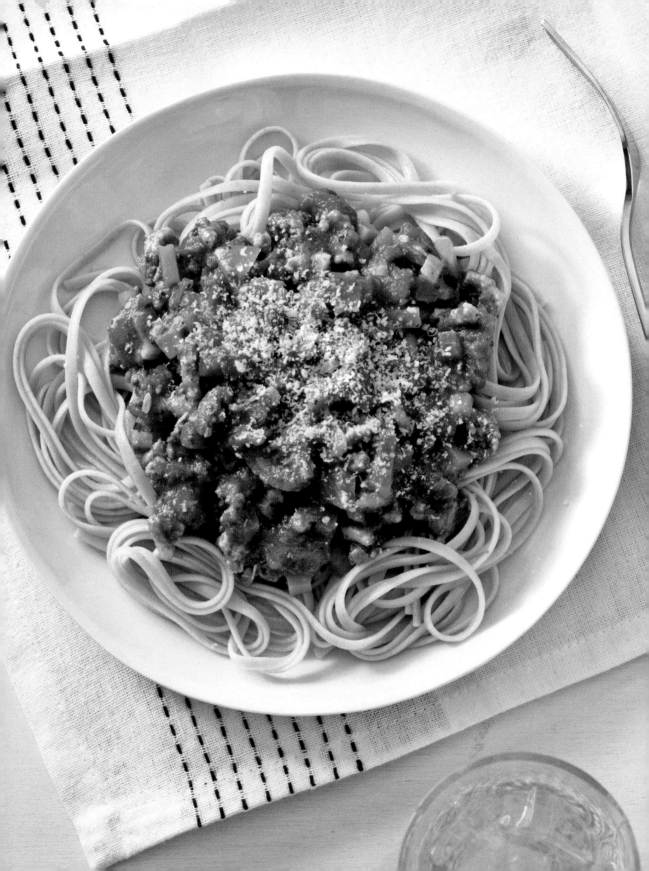

Pasta with Bolognese Sauce

SERVES 6

½ pound extra-lean ground beef

1 cup chopped onions

½ teaspoon vegetable oil

½ pound lean ground pork

½ cup chopped carrot

3 cloves garlic, minced

2 cans (14½ ounces each) no-salt-added diced tomatoes

¾ cup reduced-sodium beef broth or reduced-sodium chicken broth

¼ cup tomato paste

1½ teaspoons dried basil leaves

½ teaspoon dried oregano leaves

½ teaspoon crushed red pepper

½ teaspoon fennel seeds, crushed

¼ teaspoon salt

¼ cup whole milk

12 ounces whole-wheat dried pasta such as linguine or spaghetti

⅓ cup grated Parmesan cheese (optional)

Here, lean ground beef and pork blend in hearty sauce for whole-grain pasta. In an old Italian trick, a splash of milk stirred into the sauce before serving enhances the flavor.

1 In nonstick Dutch oven, cook beef and onions in oil over medium-high heat until beef is no longer pink, stirring to break up beef. Remove from Dutch oven.

2 In same Dutch oven cook pork, carrot and garlic until pork is no longer pink, stirring to break up pork. Drain off any fat. Return beef and onion to Dutch oven.

3 Stir in undrained tomatoes, broth, tomato paste, basil, oregano, red pepper, fennel and salt. Bring to boiling. Reduce heat. Simmer, uncovered, about 25 minutes or until desired consistency, stirring occasionally. Stir in milk. Cook about 1 minute to heat through.

4 Meanwhile, cook pasta according to package directions. Drain. Serve sauce over pasta. Sprinkle with Parmesan cheese, if desired.

Here's to your health

The pasta aisles of supermarkets and health food stores offer you a wide variety of healthful dried pasta choices. In addition to the whole-wheat pasta called for, look for pasta with added bran and fiber; pasta containing flax seeds, containing omega-3 fatty acids; fat-free dried egg noodles made with egg whites only; pasta made with hearty grains such as spelt (an ancient form of wheat) and quinoa; and gluten-free pasta made from such ingredients as brown rice, potatoes or soy.

NUTRITION FACTS PER SERVING Calories: 430; **Calories from Fat:** 110; **Total Fat:** 13g; **Saturated Fat:** 4.5g; **Trans Fat:** 0g; **Cholesterol:** 50mg; **Sodium:** 340mg; **Total Carbohydrate:** 56g; **Dietary Fiber:** 9g; **Sugars:** 10g; **Protein:** 27g

Sautéed Veal
WITH Balsamic Sauce

12 ounces veal scaloppini, cut ¼ inch thick

½ teaspoon coarsely ground black pepper

2 teaspoons vegetable oil

2 tablespoons finely chopped shallot

½ cup good-quality balsamic vinegar

2 tablespoons honey

2 tablespoons chopped fresh parsley (optional)

Tender veal cooks rapidly when it's cut into thin scallops. Simple seasonings, plus a sauce quickly made in the pan after sautéing, highlight the meat's natural sweet flavor.

1 Rub both sides of veal with pepper.

2 In large nonstick skillet heat 1 teaspoon of the oil over medium-high heat. Add half of the veal. Cook, uncovered, for 2 to 3 minutes or until no longer pink, turning once. Transfer to serving platter. Keep warm. Repeat with the remaining oil and remaining veal.

3 Add shallot to skillet. Cook about 30 seconds or until tender. Stir in vinegar and honey. Bring to boiling, scraping up any browned bits. Gently boil, uncovered, about 4 minutes or until liquid is reduced by half. Spoon over veal. Sprinkle with parsley (if desired).

NUTRITION FACTS PER SERVING Calories: 190; **Calories from Fat:** 45; **Total Fat:** 5g; **Saturated Fat:** 1g; **Trans Fat:** 0g; **Cholesterol:** 70mg; **Sodium:** 85mg; **Total Carbohydrate:** 15g; **Dietary Fiber:** 0g; **Sugars:** 13g; **Protein:** 17g

Pork Chops
WITH Pomegranate Glaze

SERVES 4

¾ teaspoon salt

¾ teaspoon ground cinnamon

¾ teaspoon pepper

6 boneless pork loin chops, cut about 1 inch thick

Cooking spray

1½ cups pomegranate juice

2 tablespoons sugar

4 tablespoons sliced green onions

Here, pomegranate juice, reduced to a syrup with just a touch of sugar, becomes an intriguing, peppery glaze for quickly seared pork chops.

1 In small bowl stir together salt, cinnamon and pepper. Rub on both sides of pork chops.

2 In large nonstick skillet coated with cooking spray, cook pork chops over medium heat for 7 to 10 minutes or until lightly browned and nearly done, turning once. Remove from skillet. Keep warm.

3 In same skillet combine pomegranate juice and sugar. Bring to boiling. Boil, uncovered, for 2 to 3 minutes or until mixture is reduced by half. Return pork chops to skillet. Cook, uncovered, about 1 minute more or until sauce thickens slightly and pork chops are done. Transfer to serving plates. Sprinkle with onions.

Make it a meal

Add these delicious side dishes to each serving to create a full meal (total additional calories: 459 per serving)

- 1 cup broccoli florets and ¼ cup chopped or slivered red bell peppers steamed together
- 8 ounces roasted new red potatoes
- 1 cup raspberries with ½ cup vanilla nonfat frozen yogurt
- Sparkling water with lime wedge

NUTRITION FACTS PER SERVING Calories: 310; **Calories from Fat:** 70; **Total Fat:** 8g; **Saturated Fat:** 2.5g; **Trans Fat:** 0g; **Cholesterol:** 140mg; **Sodium:** 420mg; **Total Carbohydrate:** 14g; **Dietary Fiber:** 0g; **Sugars:** 13g; **Protein:** 45g

Moroccan Lamb and Chickpea Stew

SERVES 8

1½ pounds boneless
leg of lamb

1 teaspoon ground
coriander

1 teaspoon ground cumin

1 teaspoon ground ginger

1 teaspoon ground
cinnamon

½ teaspoon salt

⅛ teaspoon
cayenne pepper

1 medium onion, cut
into thin wedges

3 cloves garlic, minced

2 teaspoons vegetable oil

1 can (28 ounces)
crushed tomatoes

1 can (15 ounces)
no-salt-added chickpeas,
rinsed and drained

1½ cups reduced-sodium
beef broth

1½ cups sliced carrots

1 cup dried apricot halves

½ teaspoon sugar

4 cups hot cooked
instant couscous,
prepared following
package directions

Traditional North African aromatic seasonings give this lamb-and-vegetable stew an enticing, full-bodied flavor. The recipe also works well with lean, well-trimmed beef sirloin.

1 Trim fat from meat. Cut into 1- to 1½-inch pieces. In shallow dish combine coriander, cumin, ginger, cinnamon, salt and cayenne pepper. Coat meat with spice mixture. Set aside.

2 In nonstick Dutch oven cook onion and garlic in 1 teaspoon of the oil over medium-high heat until tender. Remove from Dutch oven. Add remaining oil to pan. Quickly brown meat pieces, half at a time, in hot oil. Return all meat and onion mixture to Dutch oven.

3 Add undrained tomatoes, chickpeas, broth, carrots, apricots and sugar. Bring to boiling. Reduce heat. Simmer, covered, about 45 minutes, or until meat and vegetables are tender.

4 Spoon couscous into serving bowls. Ladle stew over couscous.

Here's to your health

How does this recipe deliver such a generous amount of protein with just 3 ounces of meat per person? Chickpeas are the answer. Part of the meat and beans food group in MyPyramid, they're high in protein as well as being a source of dietary fiber and other nutrients including folic acid and iron.

NUTRITION FACTS PER SERVING Calories: 420; **Calories from Fat:** 120; **Total Fat:** 14g; **Saturated Fat:** 6g; **Trans Fat:** 0g; **Cholesterol:** 55mg; **Sodium:** 410mg; **Total Carbohydrate:** 50g; **Dietary Fiber:** 7g; **Sugars:** 15g; **Protein:** 25g

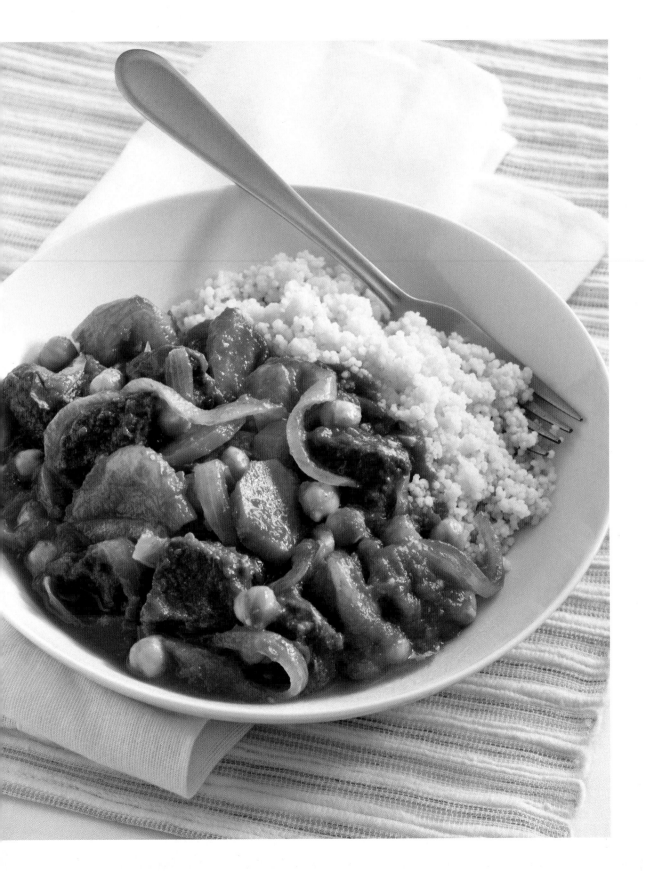

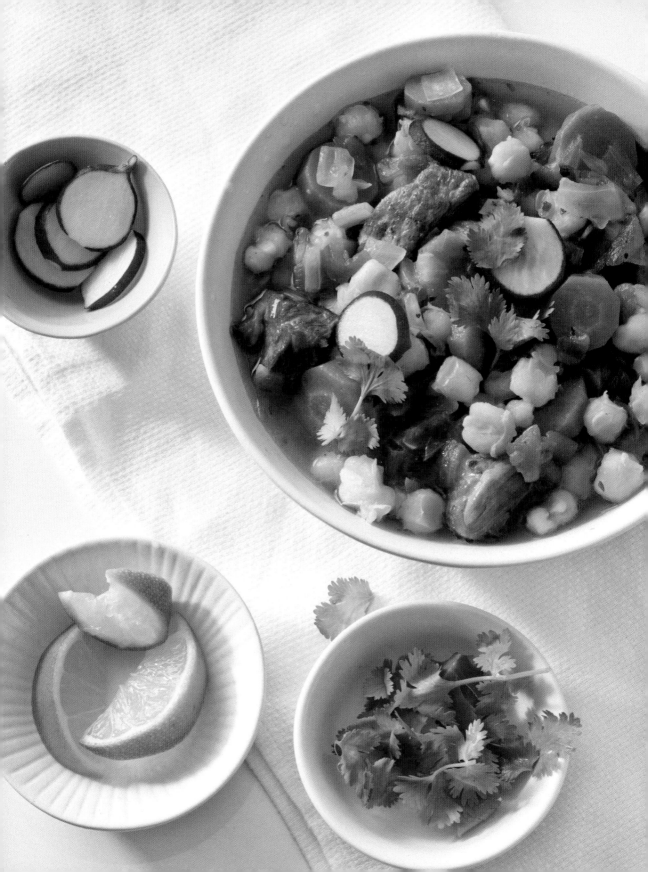

Pork Posole

1¼ pounds lean pork stew meat, trimmed and cut into 1-inch pieces

2 teaspoons vegetable oil

1 cup chopped onion

2 cloves garlic, minced

3 cups reduced-sodium chicken broth

1½ cups sliced carrots

1½ teaspoons dried oregano leaves

½ teaspoon ground cumin

¼ teaspoon crushed red pepper

2 cans (15½ ounces each) golden hominy, drained

1 can (4 ounces) chopped green chilies, drained

⅓ cup chopped fresh cilantro

⅓ cup sliced radishes

Lime wedges (optional)

Part stew, part soup, part grain course and part meat dish, this combination of golden hominy and lean pork with zesty seasonings is a hearty Mexican-style favorite.

1 In nonstick Dutch oven quickly brown pork, half at a time, in 1 teaspoon of the oil over medium-high heat. Remove all pork from Dutch oven and drain off any fat. Add remaining oil to Dutch oven. Stir in onion and garlic. Cook over medium heat until tender. Return all pork to Dutch oven.

2 Stir in broth, carrots, oregano, cumin and red pepper. Bring to boiling. Reduce heat. Simmer, covered, for 30 minutes. Stir in hominy and green chilies. Return to boiling. Reduce heat. Simmer, covered, about 5 minutes more or until heated through and pork is tender.

3 Ladle into serving bowls. Pass bowls of cilantro, radishes and lime wedges (if desired) for garnishing to taste.

Here's to your health

Pork is the traditional meat for making posole, but you can easily substitute another protein if you prefer. This recipe will also work well with lean beef or lamb stew meat, or with chunks of boneless, skinless turkey thighs or chicken thighs. You can also offer different options for topping individual servings at the table, such as thinly shredded cabbage and finely chopped sweet yellow or red onion.

NUTRITION FACTS PER SERVING **Calories:** 270; **Calories from Fat:** 60; **Total Fat:** 7g; **Saturated Fat:** 2g; **Trans Fat:** 0g; **Cholesterol:** 60mg; **Sodium:** 760mg; **Total Carbohydrate:** 30g; **Dietary Fiber:** 6g; **Sugars:** 4g; **Protein:** 25g

Asian Pork, Noodle AND Bok Choy Stir-Fry

SERVES 4

4 ounces dried whole-wheat spaghetti

¾ pound pork tenderloin

¼ cup water

2 tablespoons reduced-sodium soy sauce

2 tablespoons hot-style chili-garlic sauce

1 tablespoon oyster sauce

1 teaspoon cornstarch

2 teaspoons vegetable oil

½ medium onion, cut into slivers

1 tablespoon grated fresh ginger

4 cups thinly sliced bok choy

1½ cups matchstick-cut carrots

The lively flavors of this dish are inspired by the cuisines of several Asian nations, all of which make frequent use of quick, easy, low-fat stir-frying.

1 Cook spaghetti according to package directions. Drain. Thoroughly rinse with cold water. Drain well. Set aside.

2 Meanwhile, trim any fat from pork tenderloin. Cut into thin, bite-size pieces. Set aside.

3 In small bowl stir together water, soy sauce, chili sauce, oyster sauce and cornstarch. Set aside.

4 In nonstick wok or large nonstick skillet, heat 1 teaspoon of the oil over high heat. Add onion. Stir-fry for 3 minutes. Add ginger. Stir-fry for 30 seconds. Add bok choy and carrots. Stir-fry for 2 to 3 minutes or until vegetables are crisp-tender. Remove from wok.

5 Add remaining oil to wok. Add pork. Stir-fry about 3 minutes or until no longer pink. Stir oyster sauce mixture. Add to wok. Cook and stir until boiling. Return vegetables to wok. Add spaghetti. Cook and gently toss until heated through and combined.

NUTRITION FACTS PER SERVING Calories: 270; **Calories from Fat:** 50; **Total Fat:** 6g; **Saturated Fat:** 1.5g; **Trans Fat:** 0g; **Cholesterol:** 55mg; **Sodium:** 690mg; **Total Carbohydrate:** 31g; **Dietary Fiber:** 6g; **Sugars:** 5g; **Protein:** 24g

Pork Stew with Root Vegetables and Dried Fruits

SERVES 6

1 medium onion, halved and thinly sliced

2 teaspoons vegetable oil

1½ pounds pork tenderloin, trimmed of fat and cut into 1½-inch pieces

4 medium carrots, cut into 1-inch pieces

4 medium parsnips, cut into 1-inch pieces

1 cup apple juice

1 cup dried apricot halves

1 cup pitted prunes

½ cup reduced-sodium chicken broth

½ teaspoon salt

½ teaspoon dried thyme leaves

¼ teaspoon dried sage leaves

⅛ teaspoon allspice

Tangy dried fruit and robust root vegetables have as much of a presence as the chunks of lean, tender pork in this savory-sweet stew. It's perfect for a chilly autumn or winter evening.

1 In nonstick Dutch oven cook onion in 1 teaspoon of the oil over medium heat until tender, stirring occasionally. Remove onion from Dutch oven and set aside.

2 Add remaining oil to same Dutch oven. Quickly brown pork, half at a time, over medium-high heat. Return onion and all pork to Dutch oven. Stir in carrots, parsnips, apple juice, apricots, prunes, broth, salt, thyme, sage and allspice. Bring to boiling. Reduce heat.

3 Simmer, covered, for 35 to 40 minutes or until meat and vegetables are tender. Ladle into serving bowls.

Make it a meal

Add these delicious side dishes to each serving to create a full meal (total additional calories: 388 per serving)

- 1 cup steamed brown rice garnished with 1 tablespoon thinly sliced green onions
- Gingered Pear and Cranberry Crumble (page 215)
- Unsweetened iced tea with lemon wedge

NUTRITION FACTS PER SERVING Calories: 350; Calories from Fat: 40; **Total Fat:** 4.5g; **Saturated Fat:** 1g; **Trans Fat:** 0g; **Cholesterol:** 75mg; **Sodium:** 310mg; **Total Carbohydrate:** 54g; **Dietary Fiber:** 8g; **Sugars:** 35g; **Protein:** 27g

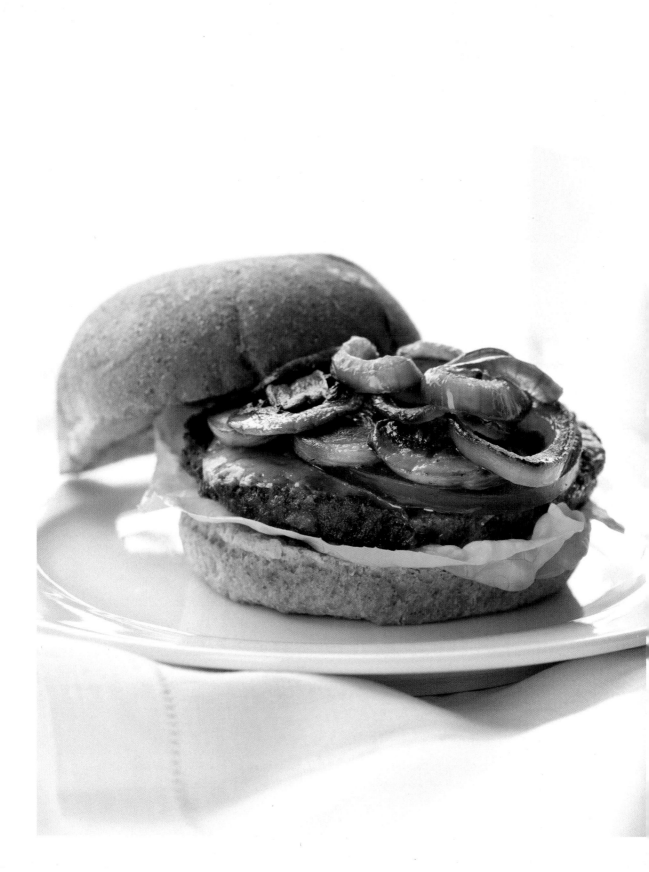

Vegetarian Main Dishes

Greek-Style Spaghetti Squash 178

Cheese Ravioli with Chunky Marinara Sauce 181

Broccoli and Tofu Stir-Fry 182

Cheese-and-Spinach Pie 183

Southwestern Vegetarian Chili 184

Vegetable Fried Rice 186

Curried Sweet Potato Patties 187

Veggie Burgers with Gruyère and Mushrooms 189

Veggie Bacon Avocado Sandwiches 190

Veggie Patties with Salsa 191

Greek-Style Spaghetti Squash

SERVES 4

One 2½- to 3-pound
spaghetti squash

1 cup reduced-sodium
chicken broth

1 cup chopped onion

3 cloves garlic, minced

2 cans (14½ ounces
each) no-salt-added
diced tomatoes

⅓ cup tomato paste

1½ teaspoons
dried marjoram

½ teaspoon salt

½ teaspoon cinnamon

¼ teaspoon nutmeg

6 cups fresh baby spinach

⅓ cup crumbled reduced-
fat feta cheese

Spaghetti squash gets its name because, when cooked, its flesh separates into strands that look like golden spaghetti. It is equally delicious served with your favorite pasta sauce.

1 Preheat oven to 350°F.

2 Halve squash lengthwise. Scoop out seeds. Place squash halves, cut side down, in 13 x 9 x 2-inch baking dish. Bake in preheated oven for 40 to 60 minutes or until tender.

3 Meanwhile, in large saucepan combine broth, onion and garlic. Bring to boiling. Reduce heat. Simmer, covered, for 5 minutes. Stir in undrained tomatoes, tomato paste, marjoram, salt, cinnamon and nutmeg. Bring to boiling. Reduce heat. Simmer, uncovered, for 7 to 12 minutes or until desired consistency.

4 Using two forks, scrape pulp from squash, letting it separate into spaghetti-like strings, onto serving platter. Cover platter with foil and keep squash warm.

5 Stir spinach into tomato mixture just until wilted. Spoon over spaghetti squash. Sprinkle with feta cheese.

NUTRITION FACTS PER SERVING Calories: 190; Calories from Fat: 15; Total Fat: 1.5g; Saturated Fat: 1g; Trans Fat: 0g; Cholesterol: 5mg; Sodium: 670mg; Total Carbohydrate: 38g; Dietary Fiber: 8g; Sugars: 16g; Protein: 18g

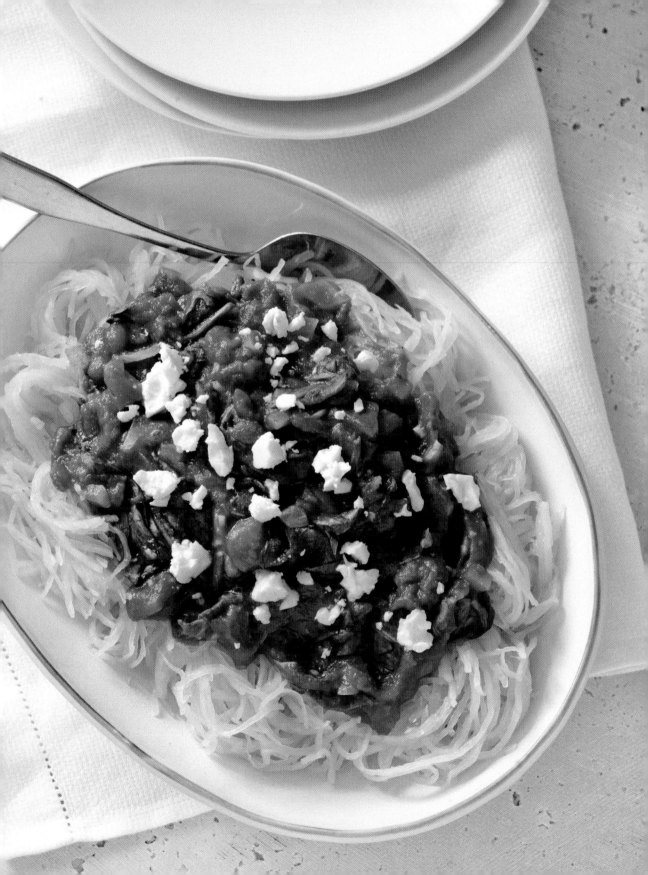

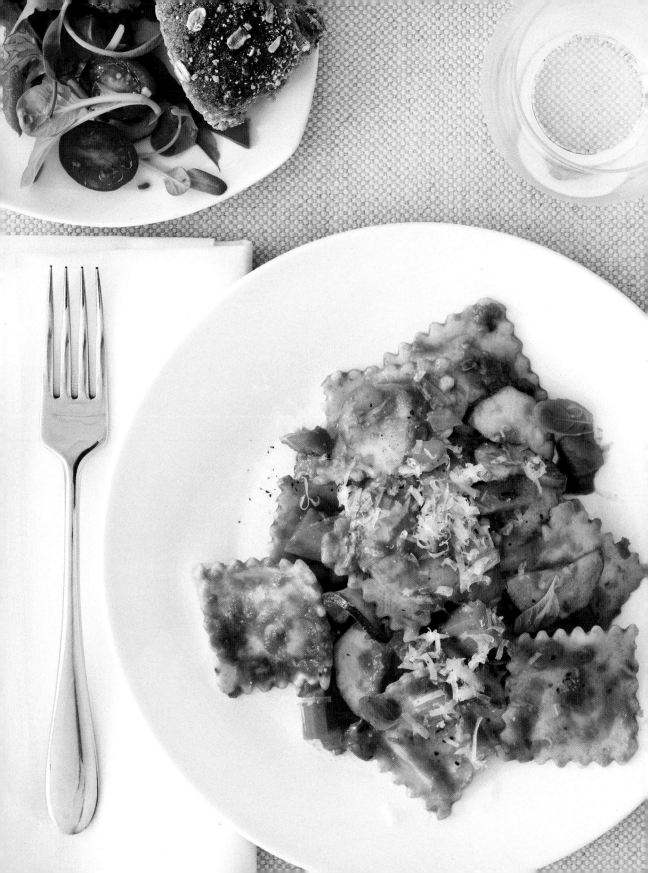

Cheese Ravioli
with Chunky Marinara Sauce

6 cups refrigerated
reduced-fat four-cheese
ravioli (about 1 pound
uncooked)

4 cups water

1 cup coarsely
chopped carrots

¼ cup chopped onion

3 cups prepared
marinara sauce

1 medium zucchini, halved
lengthwise and sliced

½ teaspoon fennel
seeds, crushed

4 teaspoons finely
shredded Parmesan
cheese (optional)

4 teaspoons slivered
fresh basil (optional)

Many well-stocked supermarkets carry ravioli with reduced-fat cheese filling in the refrigerated case. Or, substitute fresh pasta and grate some low-fat cheese over the sauce.

1 Cook ravioli according to package directions.

2 Meanwhile, in small saucepan combine water, carrot and onion. Bring to boiling. Reduce heat. Simmer, uncovered, for 2 minutes. Drain well. Return vegetables to saucepan. Stir in marinara sauce, zucchini and fennel. Bring to boiling. Reduce heat. Simmer, covered, for 1 minute. Remove lid. Simmer, uncovered, for 1 to 3 minutes more or until desired consistency.

3 Arrange ravioli on serving plates. Spoon marinara mixture on top. Sprinkle with cheese and basil (if desired).

Make it a meal

Add these delicious side dishes to each serving to create a full meal (total additional calories: 150 per serving)

- Tossed salad with 2 tablespoons fat-free salad dressing
- 1 multigrain Italian or French roll
- Sparkling water with lime wedge

NUTRITION FACTS PER SERVING Calories: 490; Calories from Fat: 130; Total Fat: 15g; Saturated Fat: 6g; Trans Fat: 0g; Cholesterol: 60mg; Sodium: 1490mg; Total Carbohydrate: 69g; Dietary Fiber: 8g; Sugars: 16g; Protein: 21g

Broccoli AND Tofu Stir-Fry

¼ cup reduced-sodium vegetable or chicken broth

3 tablespoons reduced-sodium soy sauce

1 tablespoon rice vinegar

2 teaspoons grated fresh ginger

2 teaspoons cornstarch

¼ teaspoon crushed red pepper

1½ teaspoons vegetable oil

4 cloves garlic, minced

4 cups broccoli florets

1 cup chopped red bell pepper

8 ounces extra-firm tofu, drained and cut into ½-inch pieces

2 cups hot cooked brown rice

2 tablespoons lightly salted dry-roasted peanuts (optional)

As flavorful and colorful as it is rich in iron and other nutrients, this stir-fry is a perfect example of a vegetarian main dish that even dedicated meat eaters will enjoy.

1 In small bowl stir together broth, soy sauce, vinegar, ginger, cornstarch and crushed red pepper. Set aside.

2 In nonstick wok or large nonstick skillet, heat oil over high heat. Add garlic. Stir-fry for 30 seconds. Add broccoli and bell pepper. Stir-fry for 3 to 4 minutes or until vegetables are crisp-tender. Remove from wok.

3 Stir broth mixture. Add to wok. Cook, stirring frequently, until boiling. Gently stir in vegetables and tofu. Cook and stir for 1 to 2 minutes or until heated through. Divide rice among individual plates or bowls. Spoon vegetables and tofu over rice. Sprinkle with peanuts (if desired) and serve.

NUTRITION FACTS PER SERVING Calories: 240; **Calories from Fat:** 50; **Total Fat:** 6g; **Saturated Fat:** 0g; **Trans Fat:** 0g; **Cholesterol:** 0mg; **Sodium:** 490mg; **Total Carbohydrate:** 35g; **Dietary Fiber:** 6g; **Sugars:** 3g; **Protein:** 12g

Cheese-and-Spinach Pie

SERVES 8

1 package (11 ounces) refrigerated soft bread stick dough

Cooking spray

4 egg whites or ½ cup refrigerated fat-free egg product

1 cup evaporated fat-free milk

1 tablespoon all-purpose flour

¼ teaspoon salt

½ teaspoon dry mustard

½ teaspoon Italian seasoning

2 cups **Kellogg's® Special K®** cereal (crushed to 1 cup)

1 cup cooked brown rice

1 cup chopped seeded tomatoes

1 package (10 ounces) frozen chopped spinach, thawed and thoroughly drained

¼ cup sliced green onions

½ cup crumbled feta cheese

½ cup shredded mozzarella cheese

Convenience foods and everyday pantry ingredients, including **Special K** cereal, combine in this easy recipe for a healthy and filling vegetarian main course.

1 Preheat oven to 350°F.

2 Arrange dough in circle on lightly floured work surface. Let rest 10 minutes. With rolling pin, flatten dough into 12-inch circle, sealing holes. Place in 10-inch pie plate coated with cooking spray. Set aside.

3 In medium mixing bowl, combine egg whites, milk, flour, salt, mustard and Italian seasoning. Set aside.

4 Spread remaining ingredients evenly in crust, in order listed. Pour egg mixture over ingredients.

5 Bake in preheated oven about 45 minutes or until center is set. Let cool 10 minutes before cutting into wedges and serving.

Make it a meal

Add these delicious side dishes to each serving to create a full meal (total additional calories: 221 per serving)

- 1 cup watercress leaves and ¼ medium red bell pepper cut into thin strips
- Toss with 2 tablespoons bottled fat-free Italian dressing
- 1 medium multigrain dinner roll
- 1 cup diced fresh pineapple drizzled with 1 teaspoon honey

NUTRITION FACTS PER SERVING Calories: 260; Calories from Fat: 60; **Total Fat:** 6g; **Saturated Fat:** 3g; **Trans Fat:** 0g; **Cholesterol:** 14mg; **Sodium:** 820mg; **Total Carbohydrate:** 38g; **Dietary Fiber:** 2g; **Sugars:** 3g; **Protein:** 14g

Southwestern Vegetarian Chili

SERVES 4

Cooking spray

1 cup chopped onions

4 cloves garlic, minced

2 to 4 teaspoons
chili powder

4 cans (10 ounces each)
diced tomatoes and mild
green chili

2 cups kidney beans,
rinsed and drained

1 cup no-salt-added
tomato sauce

4 tablespoons shredded
reduced-fat cheddar
cheese

4 tablespoons fat-free
sour cream

4 tablespoons sliced
green onions

Chili lovers will enjoy this healthy vegetarian version. For a meaty variation, cook ½ pound extra-lean ground turkey along with the onions and garlic and use 1 cup kidney beans.

1 In medium saucepan coated with cooking spray cook and stir onions and garlic over medium heat about 3 minutes or until tender.

2 Stir in chili powder. Cook and stir for 30 seconds. Add undrained tomatoes, beans and tomato sauce. Bring to boiling. Reduce heat. Simmer, uncovered, for 3 to 5 minutes or until desired consistency. Ladle into bowls. Top with cheese, sour cream and onions.

Make it a meal

Add these delicious side dishes to each serving to create a full meal (total additional calories: 309 per serving)

- 24 **Special K** Multi-Grain Crackers

- 6 ounces low-fat peach yogurt topped with 2 to 4 tablespoons fresh blueberries

- Unsweetened iced tea with lemon wedge

NUTRITION FACTS PER SERVING **Calories:** 250; **Calories from Fat:** 15; **Total Fat:** 1.5g; **Saturated Fat:** 0g; **Trans Fat:** 0g; **Cholesterol:** 0mg; **Sodium:** 440mg; **Total Carbohydrate:** 45g; **Dietary Fiber:** 11g; **Sugars:** 16g; **Protein:** 12g

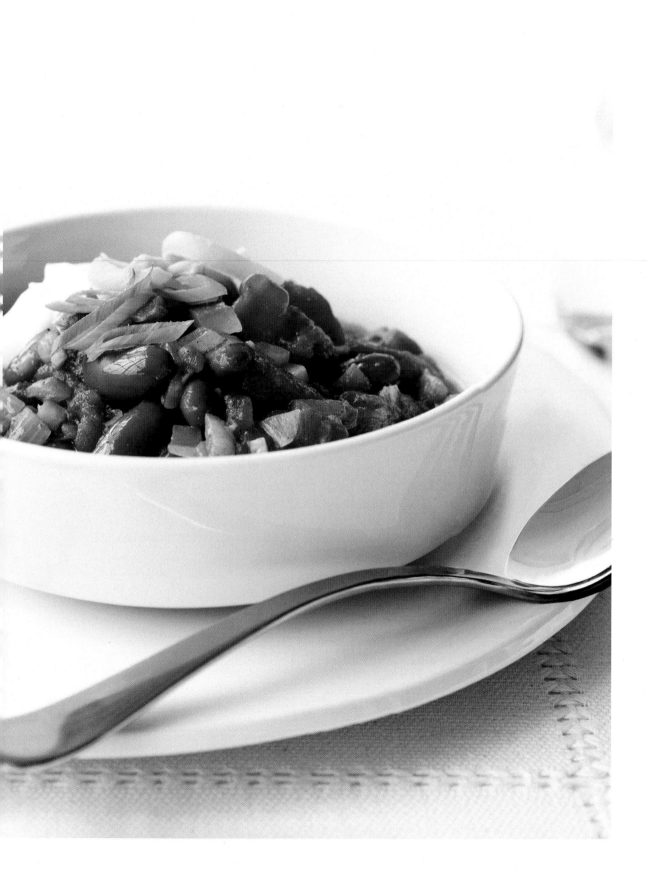

Vegetable Fried Rice

¾ cup refrigerated fat-free egg product

3 tablespoons reduced-sodium soy sauce

1 tablespoon vegetable oil

2 teaspoons grated fresh ginger

2 cloves garlic, minced

2 cups thinly sliced bok choy

1 cup sliced carrots

¾ cup chopped red bell pepper

4 green onions, cut into 1-inch pieces

3 cups cold cooked brown rice

4 teaspoons hoisin sauce

1 tablespoon rice vinegar

In this version of Chinese-style fried rice, a nonstick wok and fat-free egg product produce a vegetarian main dish that is not only lower in fat but higher in fiber than the original.

1 In small mixing bowl combine egg product and 1 tablespoon of the soy sauce. Set aside.

2 In nonstick wok or large nonstick skillet, heat 2 teaspoons of oil over medium heat. Add egg mixture. Cook, stirring, for 2 to 3 minutes or until set. Remove from wok. Cut up large pieces of egg. Set aside.

3 Add remaining oil to wok. Heat over high heat. Add ginger and garlic. Stir-fry for 30 seconds. Add bok choy, carrots, bell pepper and onions. Stir-fry for 3 to 4 minutes or until crisp-tender. Stir in remaining soy sauce, brown rice, hoisin sauce and vinegar. Stir-fry about 2 minutes or until heated through. Add egg. Cook, stirring occasionally, until heated through.

Make it your own

You have lots of flexibility preparing this dish to your taste:

- Add ¼ cup minced onion with the garlic and ginger. Or, add ½ teaspoon toasted sesame oil with the hoisin

- Substitute similar quantities of other vegetables such as sliced mushrooms, small broccoli or cauliflower florets or small snow peas

- Add cubes of well-drained firm tofu to the vegetables at the last minute of cooking. Add small pieces of cooked chicken, cooked small shrimp or flaked cooked seafood

NUTRITION FACTS PER SERVING Calories: 270; **Calories from Fat:** 45; **Total Fat:** 5g; **Saturated Fat:** 0.5g; **Trans Fat:** 0g; **Cholesterol:** 0mg; **Sodium:** 690mg; **Total Carbohydrate:** 45g; **Dietary Fiber:** 5g; **Sugars:** 6g; **Protein:** 11g

Curried Sweet Potato Patties

4 medium sweet potatoes (about 2 pounds total)

1 small ripe banana

2 teaspoons orange juice

1 tablespoon curry powder

¼ teaspoon salt

⅓ cup nonfat plain yogurt

2 tablespoons peeled and seeded finely chopped cucumber

2 tablespoons sliced green onions

1 tablespoon chopped fresh mint

¼ teaspoon garlic salt

4 teaspoons vegetable oil

Indian-style raita, a seasoned mixture of yogurt, vegetables and herbs, adds both flavor and nutritional punch to these simple, skillet-browned sweet potato patties.

1 Peel potatoes. Cut into 2-inch pieces. In Dutch oven combine potatoes and enough water to cover. Bring to boiling. Reduce heat. Simmer, uncovered, for 20 to 25 minutes or until very tender. Drain well.

2 Meanwhile, use potato masher to mash banana with orange juice in large bowl. Add potatoes. Mash, adding curry powder and salt during mashing. Let stand for 20 minutes. Cover surface with plastic wrap. Refrigerate for 1 hour.

3 Meanwhile, in small bowl stir together yogurt, cucumber, onions, mint and garlic salt. Cover and refrigerate until needed.

4 Stir cold potato mixture. Shape into eight ½-inch-thick patties. In large nonstick skillet cook patties, half at a time, in 2 teaspoons of the oil over medium-high heat for 3 to 5 minutes or until light brown, turning once. Repeat with remaining patties and oil. Transfer patties to serving plates and serve with yogurt mixture.

NUTRITION FACTS PER SERVING Calories: 280; **Calories from Fat:** 45; **Total Fat:** 5g; **Saturated Fat:** 0g; **Trans Fat:** 0g; **Cholesterol:** 0mg; **Sodium:** 340mg; **Total Carbohydrate:** 55g; **Dietary Fiber:** 8g; **Sugars:** 14g; **Protein:** 5g

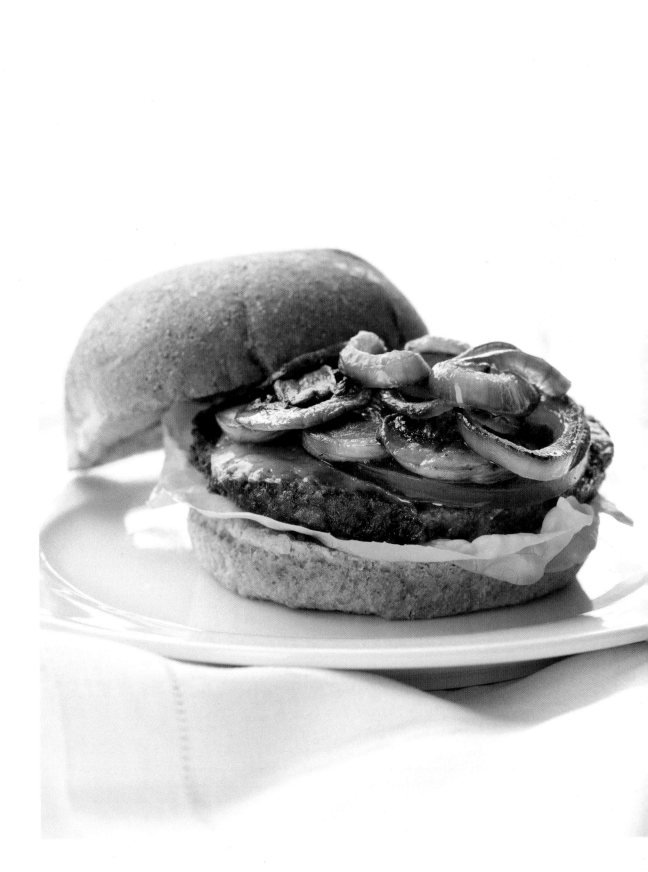

Veggie Burgers
with Gruyère and Mushrooms

4 **Morningstar Farms®
Grillers Prime®** Veggie
Burgers

4 slices Gruyère cheese
or Swiss cheese

2 teaspoons vegetable oil

2 cups sliced fresh
mushrooms

4 thin slices red onion,
separated into rings

4 lettuce leaves

4 thin slices tomato

4 whole-grain hamburger
buns, split and toasted

Occasional vegetarian meals are sensible, low-calorie options for people managing their weight. Convenient, widely available frozen veggie burgers make it easy.

1 Cook veggie burgers according to package directions. Immediately top with cheese. Let stand about 1 minute or until cheese melts.

2 Meanwhile, in small nonstick skillet heat oil over medium heat. Add mushrooms and onion. Cook, stirring frequently, for 3 to 5 minutes or until tender.

3 Place lettuce leaves, tomato slices and veggie burgers on bun bottoms. Top with mushroom mixture and bun tops.

Make it a meal

Add these delicious side dishes to each serving to create a full meal (total additional calories: 254 per serving)

- A tossed salad made from 1 to 1½ cups mixed greens, ¼ cup chopped tomato, 2 tablespoons shredded carrot, 1 tablespoon chopped red onion and 2 tablespoons fat-free salad dressing

- 1½ cups halved strawberries topped with ¼ cup low-fat vanilla yogurt and 1 to 2 teaspoons grated semisweet chocolate

- Unsweetened iced tea with lemon wedge

NUTRITION FACTS PER SERVING Calories: 420; Calories from Fat: 170; **Total Fat:** 19g; **Saturated Fat:** 5g; **Trans Fat:** 0g; **Cholesterol:** 20mg; **Sodium:** 630mg; **Total Carbohydrate:** 35g; **Dietary Fiber:** 5g; **Sugars:** 7g; **Protein:** 28g

Veggie Bacon Avocado Sandwiches

12 **Morningstar Farms®
Grillers Prime®** Veggie
Bacon Strips

2 medium ripe
avocados, seeded,
peeled and mashed
(about 1 cup total)

4 teaspoons
lemon juice

½ teaspoon salt

9 to 12 drops hot
pepper sauce

8 slices whole-grain
bread, toasted

4 lettuce leaves

16 thick slices
plum tomato

Vegetarian bacon strips, widely available frozen in supermarkets, make a healthful version of the classic BLTA sandwich
with far less fat and no cholesterol at all.

1 Cook veggie bacon strips according to package directions.

2 Meanwhile, in small bowl stir together avocados, lemon juice, salt
and pepper sauce to taste. Spread on one side of each toast slice. Place
lettuce leaf, tomato slices and bacon strips on top of half the slices.

3 Top with remaining toast slices, avocado mixture side down.
Cut sandwiches in half. Serve immediately.

Make it a meal

Add these delicious side dishes to each serving to create
a full meal (total additional calories: 306 per serving)

- ½ cup carrot sticks with 2 tablespoons ranch dressing
- 1 cup sliced or cubed fresh mango topped with
  ⅓ cup low-fat strawberry yogurt and 1 tablespoon
  low-fat granola
- Sparkling water with lime wedge

NUTRITION FACTS PER SERVING **Calories:** 360; **Calories from Fat:** 160; **Total Fat:** 17g; **Saturated Fat:** 2g; **Trans Fat:** 0g;
Cholesterol: 0mg; **Sodium:** 910mg; **Total Carbohydrate:** 39g; **Dietary Fiber:** 14g; **Sugars:** 8g; **Protein:** 13g

Veggie Patties WITH Salsa

2 cups **Kellogg's®
Special K®** cereal

1 can (15½ ounces)
kidney beans, drained

⅓ cup chopped onion

1 garlic clove, minced

1 cup coarsely chopped
mushrooms

1 can (8 ounces) sliced
water chestnuts, drained

¼ teaspoon salt

½ cup whole-kernel corn

½ cup shredded carrot

2 tablespoons
chopped cilantro

1 egg white

Cooking spray

1½ cups tomato salsa

Made with **Special K** cereal, kidney beans and vegetables, these robust patties prove how much satisfaction you can get from a vegetarian recipe packed with texture and flavor.

1 Place 1 cup of the cereal, beans, onion and garlic in food processor work bowl. Process about 1 minute or until finely chopped, scraping bowl once. Remove to large mixing bowl. Place remaining cereal, mushrooms, water chestnuts and salt in work bowl. Process about 1 minute or until finely chopped, scraping bowl once. Add to bean mixture along with corn, carrot, cilantro and egg white. Mix well.

2 Preheat nonstick skillet over medium-low heat. Spray skillet with nonstick cooking spray.

3 Using ¼-cup measure, portion vegetable mixture into hot pan. Carefully shape into patties about ½ inch thick. Cook about 3 minutes, turning once, until deep golden brown and firm. Serve patties hot with salsa.

NUTRITION FACTS PER SERVING **Calories:** 230; **Calories from Fat:** 5; **Total Fat:** 1g; **Saturated Fat:** 0g; **Trans Fat:** 0g; **Cholesterol:** 0mg; **Sodium:** 680mg; **Total Carbohydrate:** 45g; **Dietary Fiber:** 9g; **Sugars:** 3g; **Protein:** 12g

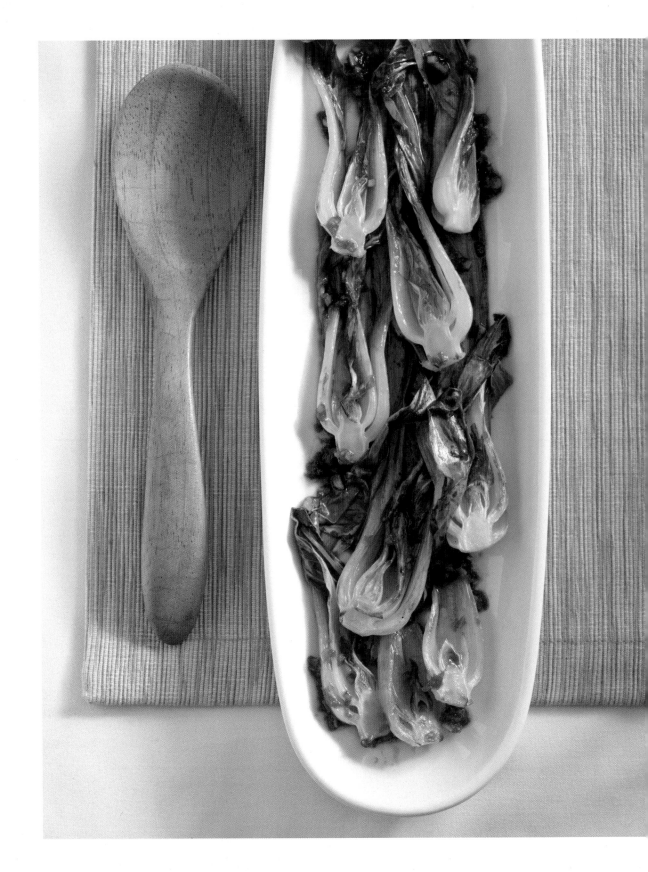

Side Dishes

Fennel AND Quinoa Oven Pilaf

½ cup chopped onion

1 clove garlic, minced

2 teaspoons vegetable oil

1 cup chopped fresh fennel bulb

1 cup uncooked quinoa, rinsed and drained

2 cups reduced-sodium chicken broth

½ teaspoon dried marjoram leaves

¼ teaspoon salt

¼ teaspoon pepper

1 cup seeded and chopped tomato

2 tablespoons chopped fresh fennel fronds

Quinoa (pronounced KEEN-wah), a grain treasured by the ancient Incas, has a subtle nutty flavor that pairs well with fennel in this easy pilaf. Try it with any saucy main dish.

1 Preheat oven to 350°F.

2 In medium nonstick saucepan cook onion and garlic in oil over medium heat until tender. Stir in fennel and quinoa. Continue cooking, stirring occasionally, for 2 minutes more.

3 Stir in chicken broth, marjoram, salt and pepper. Bring to boiling. Stir in tomato. Transfer to 2-quart casserole. Cover and bake in preheated oven about 20 minutes or until liquid is absorbed.

4 Let stand for 5 minutes. Use fork to fluff. Garnish with fennel fronds and serve immediately.

Here's to your health

Quinoa offers a wealth of nutritional benefits. Chief among these is the fact that, unlike most grains, it supplies a complete source of protein, containing all nine essential amino acids humans need to get from foods—a rarity among vegetarian protein sources. Quinoa is also a source of many other nutrients, including magnesium, manganese and copper; riboflavin (vitamin B2); and dietary fiber.

NUTRITION FACTS PER SERVING Calories: 270; Calories from Fat: 140; **Total Fat:** 16g; **Saturated Fat:** 3.5g; **Trans Fat:** 0g; **Cholesterol:** 60mg; **Sodium:** 220mg; **Total Carbohydrate:** 6g; **Dietary Fiber:** 2g; **Sugars:** 3g; **Protein:** 25g

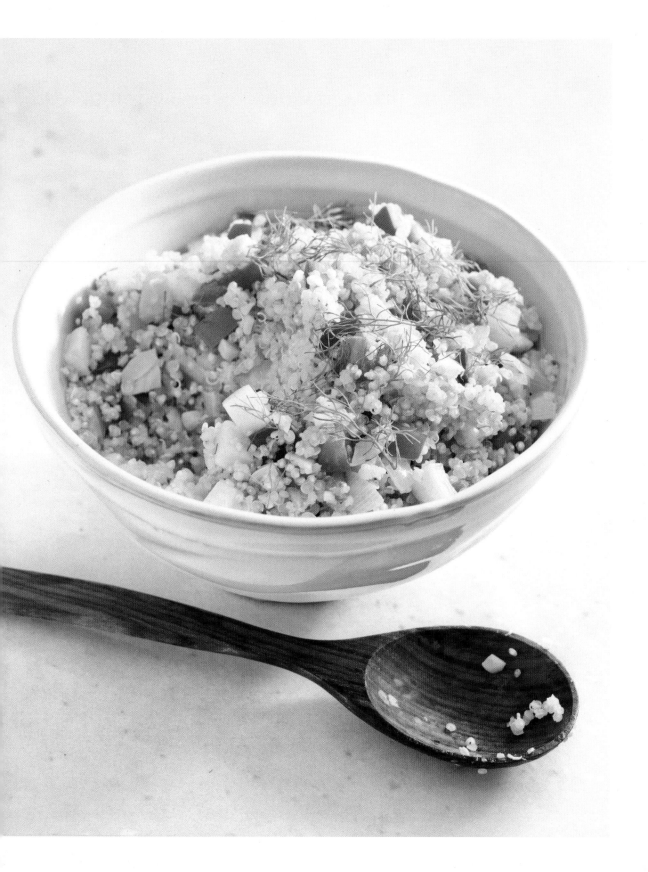

Roasted Cauliflower AND Tomatoes

1 medium head cauliflower (about 2½ pounds)

1½ cups grape tomatoes or cherry tomatoes, halved

Cooking spray

1 tablespoon reduced-sodium chicken broth

2 teaspoons vegetable oil

½ teaspoon salt

½ teaspoon turmeric

¼ teaspoon crushed red pepper

Roasting gives cauliflower a rich, nutty flavor, and golden turmeric and vibrant red tomatoes add bright bursts of taste and color. Serve this side dish with roasted meat or poultry.

1 Preheat oven to 425°F.

2 Cut cauliflower into florets. (You should have about 8 cups.) Spread cauliflower and tomatoes on 15 x 10 x 1-inch baking pan lined with foil and coated with cooking spray.

3 In small bowl stir together broth, oil, salt, turmeric and red pepper. Drizzle over cauliflower mixture. Gently stir until vegetables are coated. Bake, uncovered, in preheated oven about 40 minutes or until cauliflower is tender, stirring once after 20 minutes.

NUTRITION FACTS PER SERVING Calories: 70; Calories from Fat: 20; Total Fat: 2g; Saturated Fat: 0g; Trans Fat: 0g; Cholesterol: 0mg; Sodium: 250mg; Total Carbohydrate: 11g; Dietary Fiber: 4g; Sugars: 5g; Protein: 4g

Broccoli-Pineapple Slaw

4 cups broccoli slaw mix

½ cup shredded carrot

¼ cup finely chopped
red onion

¼ cup nonfat plain yogurt

2 tablespoons reduced-fat
mayonnaise

2 teaspoons sugar

1 teaspoon cider vinegar

¼ teaspoon salt

⅛ teaspoon celery seed

1 cup finely chopped
fresh pineapple

Tangy fresh pineapple brightens this version of vegetable slaw. For ease, look for bags of pre-shredded, ready-to-use broccoli you'll find in supermarket produce sections.

1 In large bowl combine slaw mix, carrot and red onion.

2 In small bowl whisk together yogurt, mayonnaise, sugar, vinegar, salt and celery seed. Add to slaw mixture. Toss to combine. Cover and refrigerate for 30 minutes.

3 Stir in pineapple. Serve immediately.

Here's to your health

Broccoli, featured in this recipe, is a member of a group of vegetables called brassicas, which also includes cauliflower, Brussels sprouts, kale, cabbages and bok choy and mustard greens. A source of dietary fiber, brassicas also contain vitamins A and C, as well as some calcium and iron.

NUTRITION FACTS PER SERVING Calories: 70; **Calories from Fat:** 20; **Total Fat:** 2g; **Saturated Fat:** 0g; **Trans Fat:** 0g; **Cholesterol:** 0mg; **Sodium:** 170mg; **Total Carbohydrate:** 11g; **Dietary Fiber:** 2g; **Sugars:** 6g; **Protein:** 3g

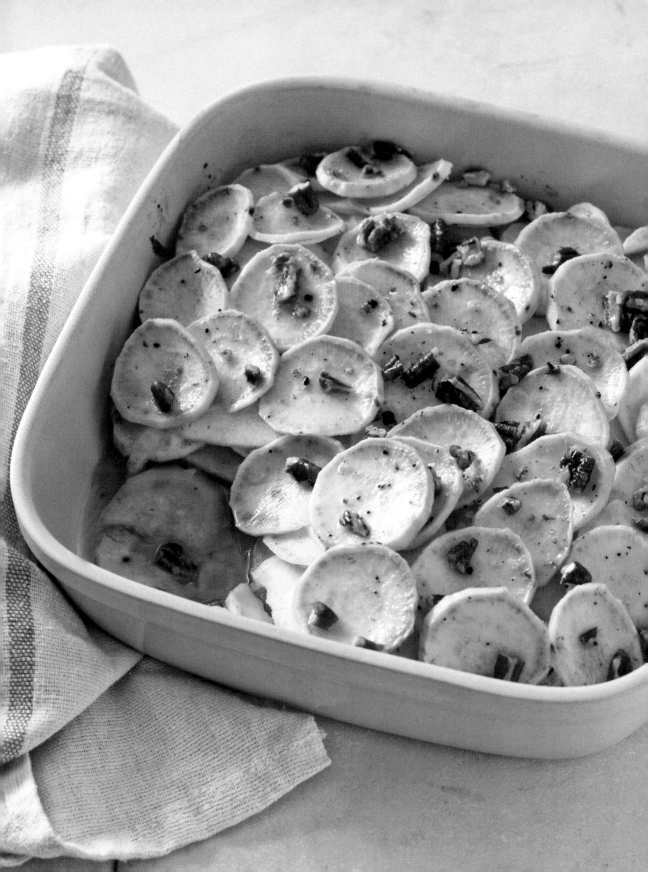

Sweet Potato, Onion
AND Apple Gratin

SERVES 6

1¾ pounds sweet potatoes, peeled and thinly sliced

⅓ cup thinly sliced onion

1 large cooking apple, cored and thinly sliced

¼ cup plus 1 tablespoon maple syrup

2 tablespoons apple juice

½ teaspoon instant chicken bouillon granules

¼ teaspoon pepper

2 tablespoons chopped pecans

Toasted pecans and a maple glaze flavor this apple, sweet potato and onion casserole. Serve this easy-to-assemble dish alongside roasted meat or poultry.

1 Preheat oven to 375°F.

2 In 8 x 8 x 2-inch baking dish, layer ⅓ of potatoes. Top with half of the onion and half of the apple. Repeat layers of ⅓ potatoes and half each of onion and apple. Top with remaining potatoes.

3 In small bowl stir together ¼ cup syrup, apple juice, bouillon granules and pepper. Drizzle over top.

4 Cover tightly with foil. Bake in preheated oven for 45 minutes. Uncover. Sprinkle with pecans and drizzle with 1 tablespoon syrup. Bake about 5 minutes longer or until pecans are toasted and vegetables are tender.

Here's to your health

Sweet potatoes are among the most healthful vegetable choices you can make. Low in calories and fat, a medium-sized sweet potato gives you about twice the amount of vitamin A you need daily and almost half the vitamin C you need. It's also a source of dietary fiber (leave the peels on in this recipe for even more fiber).

NUTRITION FACTS PER SERVING Calories: 170; **Calories from Fat:** 15; **Total Fat:** 2g; **Saturated Fat:** 0g; **Trans Fat:** 0g; **Cholesterol:** 0mg; **Sodium:** 85mg; **Total Carbohydrate:** 37g; **Dietary Fiber:** 4g; **Sugars:** 19g; **Protein:** 2g

Polenta Gratin

4 cups cold water

½ teaspoon salt

1 cup dry, slow-cooking stone-ground polenta

Cooking spray

1 cup prepared marinara sauce

2 tablespoons grated Parmesan cheese

Here, Italian-style cornmeal is baked with tangy tomato sauce and a touch of cheese for a delicious, satisfying side dish made from humble, rustic ingredients.

1 In medium saucepan bring 3 cups water and salt to boiling. Meanwhile, in small bowl whisk together polenta and 1 cup water. Slowly add polenta mixture to boiling water, stirring constantly. Cook and stir until mixture returns to boiling. Reduce heat to very low. Cover and simmer, stirring occasionally, for 20 minutes or until polenta is thick but still fluid.

2 Preheat oven to 350°F.

3 In 1-quart gratin dish or 9-inch pie plate coated with cooking spray, layer half of the polenta and ⅓ cup of the marinara sauce. Carefully spread remaining polenta over marinara sauce. Sprinkle with Parmesan cheese. Bake in preheated oven about 40 minutes or until beginning to brown.

4 Meanwhile, in small microwave-safe bowl micro-cook remaining marinara sauce at high about 1 minute or until heated through. Spoon polenta on serving plates and pass warmed sauce.

NUTRITION FACTS PER SERVING **Calories:** 80; **Calories from Fat:** 10; **Total Fat:** 1g; **Saturated Fat:** 0g; **Trans Fat:** 0g; **Cholesterol:** 0mg; **Sodium:** 300mg; **Total Carbohydrate:** 16g; **Dietary Fiber:** 2g; **Sugars:** 2g; **Protein:** 3g

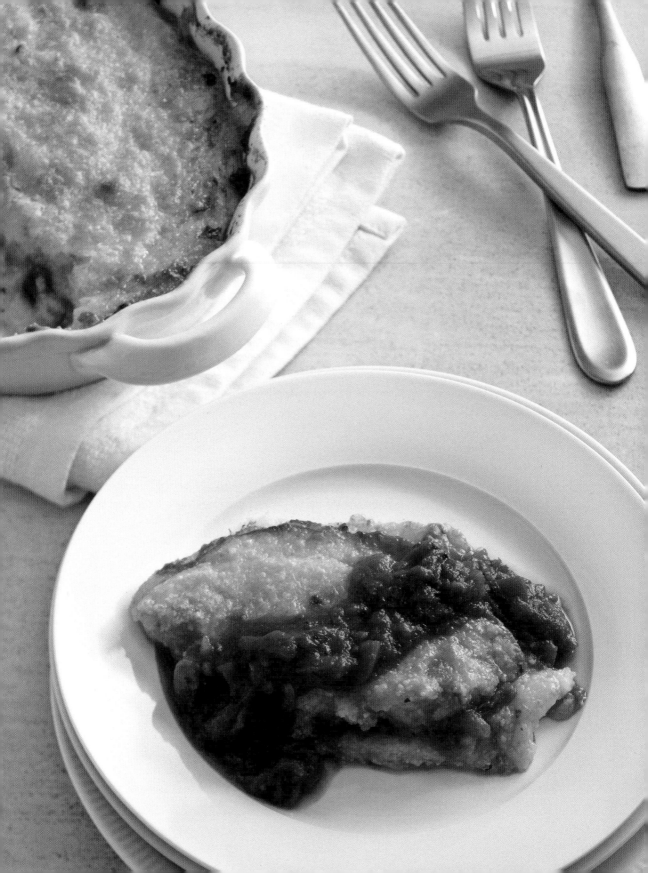

Crunchy Broccoli Bake

2 tablespoons butter

2 tablespoons flour

1 teaspoon salt

½ teaspoon freshly
ground pepper

¼ teaspoon sugar

½ teaspoon grated onion

1 cup nonfat sour cream

3 cups fresh broccoli
florets, or 2 packages
(10 ounces each)
frozen broccoli

Cooking spray

1½ cups **Kellogg's®
Special K®** cereal

1 cup finely shredded
Swiss cheese

This delicious side dish is a good alternative to plain-old broccoli. Though about 40 percent of the calories come from fat, it's because the broccoli itself is so low in calories.

1 Preheat oven to 350°F.

2 In a saucepan heat butter until melted. Stir in flour, salt, pepper, sugar, and onion. Add sour cream and stir until smooth.

3 Heat mixture, stirring constantly, until mixture starts to boil. Stir in broccoli. Pour mixture into 1½-quart baking dish lightly coated with cooking spray. Stir together cereal and cheese. Sprinkle cereal and cheese mixture over broccoli.

4 Bake in preheated oven about 20 minutes or until bubbly.

Make it your own

In this golden-brown and bubbly side dish you can change the vegetables and other ingredients to make your own versions. Try these ideas for a start:

Cauliflower gratin Substitute cauliflower florets for the broccoli and Cheddar cheese for the Swiss

Brussels sprouts gratin Cut sprouts into quarters or halves, depending on size. Add 1 teaspoon Dijon mustard to the sauce and top with mozzarella and a little grated Parmesan

Baby spinach gratin Substitute three bags (6 ounces each) prewashed baby spinach leaves for the broccoli. Substitute crumbled feta cheese for the Swiss

NUTRITION FACTS PER SERVING Calories: 190; **Calories from Fat:** 80; **Total Fat:** 9g; **Saturated Fat:** 4g; **Trans Fat:** 0g; **Cholesterol:** 15mg; **Sodium:** 590mg; **Total Carbohydrate:** 16g; **Dietary Fiber:** less than 1g; **Sugars:** 4g; **Protein:** 11g

Whipped Buttermilk Potatoes

3 pounds russet potatoes, peeled and cut into 2-inch pieces

¾ cup low-fat buttermilk

2 tablespoons butter, softened

1 teaspoon salt

¼ teaspoon pepper

Chopped fresh chives (optional)

Along with the creamy quality prized in good mashed potatoes, low-fat buttermilk also adds a pleasant, slightly tangy flavor enhanced by a touch of butter for richness.

1 In Dutch oven combine potatoes and enough water to cover. Bring to boiling. Reduce heat. Simmer, uncovered, for 15 to 20 minutes or until potatoes are very tender.

2 Meanwhile, in microwave-safe bowl combine buttermilk and butter. Micro-cook, uncovered, at high about 30 seconds or until just warm. (Do not boil.)

3 In colander drain potatoes. Return to Dutch oven. Use potato masher to mash potatoes, adding milk mixture, salt and pepper during mashing. Transfer to serving bowl. Sprinkle with chives (if desired).

NUTRITION FACTS PER SERVING Calories: 170; **Calories from Fat:** 30; **Total Fat:** 3.5g; **Saturated Fat:** 2g; **Trans Fat:** 0g; **Cholesterol:** 10mg; **Sodium:** 340mg; **Total Carbohydrate:** 32g; **Dietary Fiber:** 2g; **Sugars:** 2g; **Protein:** 5g

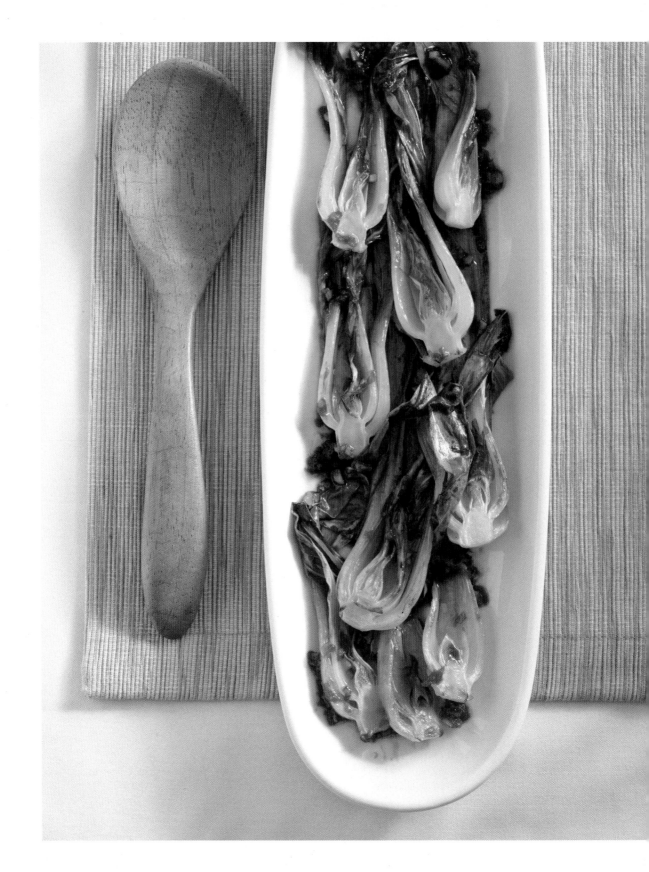

Asian-Style Braised Baby Bok Choy

2 tablespoons reduced-sodium soy sauce

1 tablespoon rice vinegar

2 teaspoons water

½ teaspoon sugar

1 pound baby bok choy or small Shanghai bok choy (about 4 heads total)

Cooking spray

2 tablespoons reduced-sodium chicken broth

2 teaspoons grated fresh ginger

2 cloves garlic, minced

Enjoying your daily servings of vegetables is easy when you combine lively seasonings such as ginger, garlic and soy sauce to flavor the mild Asian cabbage called bok choy.

1 In bowl, stir together soy sauce, vinegar, water and sugar. Set aside.

2 Trim bok choy. Halve each lengthwise. Lightly coat large nonstick skillet with cooking spray. Heat over medium heat. Add bok choy, cut side down, arranging so stems touch skillet and leaves are on top. Cook, uncovered, for 3 to 4 minutes or until beginning to brown. Turn. Drizzle with broth. Cook, covered, for 1 minute more. Use tongs to transfer bok choy to serving platter. Cover to keep warm.

3 Add ginger and garlic to skillet. Stir in soy sauce mixture. Bring to boiling. Simmer, uncovered, about 30 seconds or until beginning to thicken. Drizzle soy mixture over bok choy. Serve immediately.

Here's to your health

Look for bok choy in Asian markets—you'll also see it popping up more and more in the produce sections of supermarkets. The vegetable is a source of vitamin C, vitamin A and calcium. Like other members of the cabbage family (see page 197), it also provides antioxidants.

NUTRITION FACTS PER SERVING Calories: 225; **Calories from Fat:** 5; **Total Fat:** 0g; **Saturated Fat:** 0g; **Trans Fat:** 0g; **Cholesterol:** 0mg; **Sodium:** 380mg; **Total Carbohydrate:** 4g; **Dietary Fiber:** 1g; **Sugars:** 2g; **Protein:** 2g

Potato-Onion Casserole

¼ cup trans fat-free margarine

1½ cups **Kellogg's®
Special K®** cereal
(crushed to ¾ cup)

1 cup thinly sliced onions

4 cups thinly sliced
peeled potatoes

½ teaspoon salt

¼ cup all-purpose flour

¼ teaspoon pepper

¼ teaspoon paprika

2 cups nonfat milk

Cooking spray

Enjoy all the indulgent flavor and texture of a stuffed baked potato, with far less fat. The secret: layering potatoes and onions with creamy sauce made from nonfat milk.

1 Preheat the oven to 350°F.

2 Melt 2 tablespoons of the margarine. In medium mixing bowl, combine melted margarine with **Special K** cereal. Set aside.

3 Place onions and potatoes in medium-size saucepan. Cover with water. Add ¼ teaspoon salt. Bring to boil. Boil, uncovered, for 5 minutes. Remove from heat. Drain.

4 Melt remaining 2 tablespoons margarine in small saucepan over low heat. Stir in flour, remaining ¼ teaspoon salt, pepper and paprika. Add milk gradually, stirring until smooth. Increase heat to medium and cook until bubbly and thickened, stirring constantly. Remove from heat.

5 Arrange half the potatoes and onions in 1½-quart glass baking dish coated with cooking spray. Top with half the sauce. Repeat, ending with the sauce. Sprinkle cereal mixture evenly over the top. Bake in preheated oven about 30 minutes or until potatoes are tender.

NUTRITION FACTS PER SERVING Calories: 160; **Calories from Fat:** 50; **Total Fat:** 6g; **Saturated Fat:** 1g; **Trans Fat:** 0g; **Cholesterol:** 0mg; **Sodium:** 560mg; **Total Carbohydrate:** 21g; **Dietary Fiber:** 2g; **Sugars:** 5g; **Protein:** 5g

Roasted Winter Vegetables

Cooking spray

1 large sweet potato, peeled and cut into 1-inch pieces

1 fennel bulb, trimmed and cut into 6 wedges

2 medium red potatoes, cut into 1- to 1½-inch pieces

2 large shallots, cut into quarters

2 tablespoons vegetable oil

1 tablespoon balsamic vinegar

½ teaspoon coarse salt

½ teaspoon dried rosemary leaves

2 cloves garlic, minced

Mellow balsamic vinegar blends beautifully with fresh rosemary to flavor this colorful combination of roasted sweet potatoes, fennel, red potatoes and shallots.

1 Preheat oven to 425°F.

2 Meanwhile, on 15 x 10 x 1-inch baking pan lined with foil and coated with cooking spray, toss together sweet potato, fennel, red potatoes, shallots, oil, vinegar, salt, rosemary and garlic.

3 Bake in preheated oven about 40 minutes or until vegetables begin to brown, stirring every 10 minutes. Transfer to serving bowl.

Make it your own

Comb farmers' markets in the cooler months of the year for a wide variety of root vegetables to try. Here are suggestions for other varieties to roast using the method above:

Carrots Peel and trim whole baby carrots, or cut larger peeled and trimmed carrots into 1-inch chunks

Garlic Separate a garlic head into cloves and leave peels on. Squeeze garlic from peels after roasting

Onions Cut peeled and trimmed medium yellow onions into 8 wedges each

Parsnips Peel and trim parsnips and cut into 1-inch pieces

Turnips Peel and trim whole baby turnips, or cut larger peeled and trimmed turnips into 1-inch wedges

NUTRITION FACTS PER SERVING Calories: 150; **Calories from Fat:** 45; **Total Fat:** 5g; **Saturated Fat:** 0g; **Trans Fat:** 0g; **Cholesterol:** 0mg; **Sodium:** 230mg; **Total Carbohydrate:** 26g; **Dietary Fiber:** 3g; **Sugars:** 4g; **Protein:** 3g

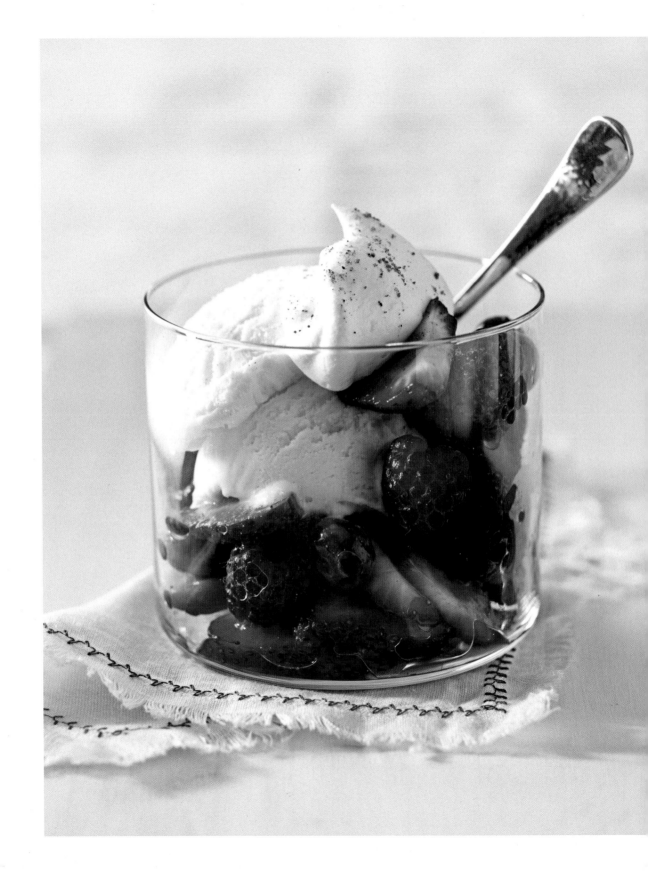

Desserts

Poached Peaches with Yogurt Cream 210

Sugar and Spice Chews 213

Baked Apples with Almond-Apricot Filling 214

Gingered Pear and Cranberry Crumble 215

Individual Mango Buckles 216

Rice Pudding with Dried Fruit 219

Streusel Dessert Squares 220

Caramel Apple Crisp 221

Red Velvet Cupcakes 222

Dark Chocolate Angel Food Cake with Raspberry Sauce 225

Easy Key Lime Mousse with Angel Food Cake 226

Cream Cheese Pie with Tropical Fruit Topping 227

Fresh Blueberry-Ginger Fool 228

Frozen Yogurt and Berry Sundaes 231

Poached Peaches with Yogurt Cream

SERVES 4

½ cup nonfat plain Greek yogurt

1 ounce reduced-fat cream cheese, softened

2 tablespoons powdered sugar

¼ teaspoon vanilla extract

⅛ teaspoon almond extract

3 tablespoons grated dark chocolate (about ½ ounce)

1½ cups cranberry-apple juice

One 2-inch piece cinnamon stick

2 medium peaches, halved, pitted and peeled; or 2 firm, ripe pears, halved and cored

A topping based on luscious nonfat Greek-style yogurt perfectly highlights tender poached summer fruit. During the cooler months, this recipe works just as well with pears.

1 In small bowl stir together yogurt, cream cheese, sugar, vanilla and almond extract. Reserve 1 tablespoon of grated chocolate. Fold remaining chocolate into yogurt mixture. Cover and refrigerate until needed.

2 In large skillet bring juice and cinnamon stick to just boiling. Carefully add peach halves. Cover and simmer for 10 to 15 minutes or until peaches are just tender. Remove peaches from poaching liquid. Continue cooking liquid, uncovered, over medium heat for 5 to 10 minutes or until reduced to ½ cup.

3 Place peach halves on 4 dessert plates. Drizzle reduced liquid over top. Spoon yogurt mixture on each. Sprinkle with reserved chocolate.

Here's to your health

Nonfat Greek-style yogurt, available in many super-markets and natural foods stores, provides rich flavor and creamy texture without fat. During its preparation, the yogurt is strained to reduce the amount of watery whey it contains. As a result, it has a thicker consistency and more intense flavor than regular yogurt, and may contain more protein per serving. Read labels to make sure the product you buy is made by this natural process rather than one that has been artificially thickened.

NUTRITION FACTS PER SERVING Calories: 140; **Calories from Fat:** 25; **Total Fat:** 3g; **Saturated Fat:** 2g; **Trans Fat:** 0g; **Cholesterol:** 5mg; **Sodium:** 55mg; **Total Carbohydrate:** 27g; **Dietary Fiber:** 2g; **Sugars:** 23g; **Protein:** 4g

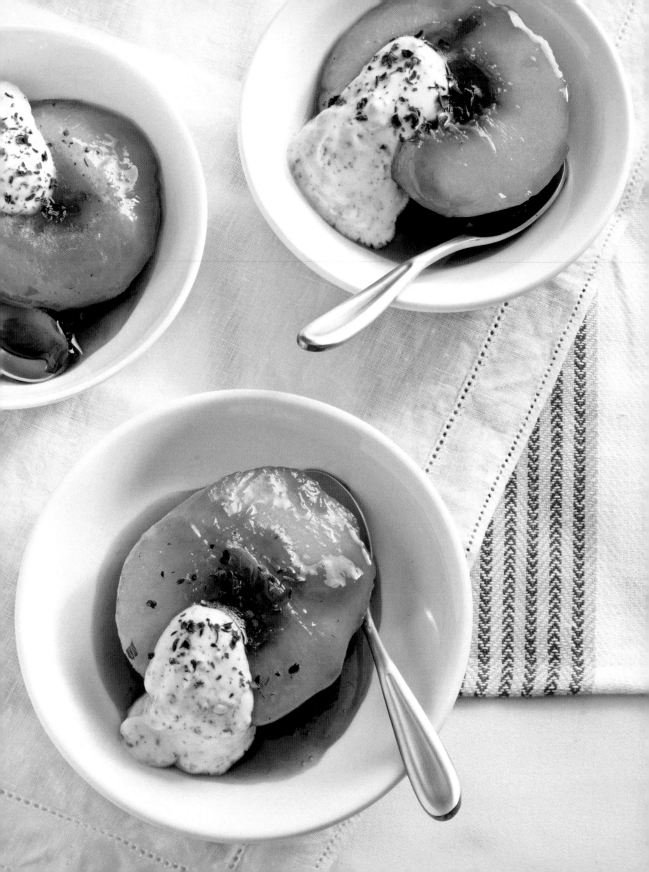

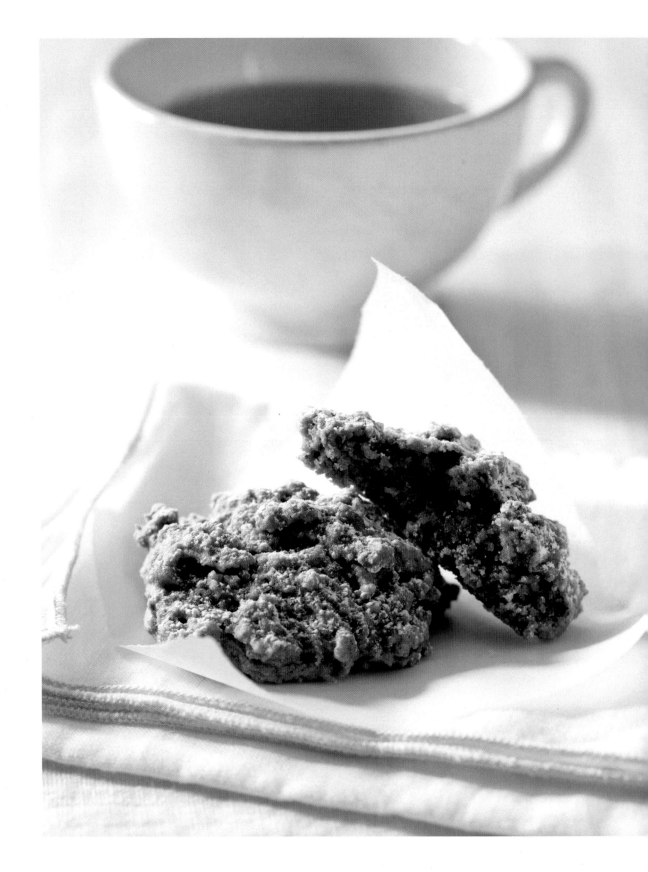

Sugar AND Spice Chews

2½ cups all-purpose flour

1 teaspoon baking soda

½ teaspoon salt

1 teaspoon apple
pie spice

2 cups **Kellogg's®
Special K®** Red
Berries cereal

1½ cups firmly packed
brown sugar

¼ cup butter or
margarine, softened

½ cup apple butter

2 egg whites

1 teaspoon vanilla

½ cup chopped nuts
(optional)

Cooking spray

Powdered sugar
(optional)

Each of these low-fat cookies made with **Special K** Red Berries cereal is so packed with great texture and flavor that two of them make a satisfying serving.

1 Preheat oven to 350°F.

2 In medium mixing bowl stir together flour, baking soda, salt and apple pie spice. Set aside.

3 In large mixing bowl, using hand-held electric mixer on medium speed, beat together **Special K** Red Berries cereal, brown sugar, butter, apple butter, egg whites, vanilla and nuts (if desired) for 2 minutes or until thoroughly combined and cereal is broken into small pieces. Add flour mixture, beating on low speed until combined. Drop by level tablespoons onto baking sheets coated with nonstick cooking spray.

4 Bake in preheated oven about 10 minutes or until edges start to brown. Cool slightly on baking sheets. Remove to wire racks and cool completely. Serve cookies dusted with powdered sugar, if desired. Store in airtight container.

NUTRITION FACTS PER SERVING Calories: 110; Calories from Fat: 15; Total Fat: 1.5g; Saturated Fat: 1g; Trans Fat: 0g; Cholesterol: 5mg; Sodium: 105mg; Total Carbohydrate: 23g; Dietary Fiber: 0g; Sugars: 14g; Protein: 1g

Baked Apples
WITH Almond-Apricot Filling

2 medium cooking apples

3 tablespoons chopped dried apricots

2 tablespoons chopped toasted almonds

2 teaspoons honey

⅛ teaspoon cinnamon

1 can (5½ ounces) apricot nectar

½ teaspoon vanilla

¼ teaspoon nutmeg

⅔ cup low-fat vanilla yogurt or low-fat lemon yogurt (optional)

Stuffed apples baked in vanilla-scented apricot nectar take on a wonderful flavor. If you wish to double the recipe, use a larger pan just big enough to hold all the apples.

1 Preheat oven to 350°F.

2 Core apples, leaving them whole. Using peeler, remove strip of peel about 1 inch wide from around middle of each apple.

3 In small bowl combine apricots, almonds, honey and cinnamon. Stand apples upright in 8 x 4 x 2-inch loaf pan. Spoon apricot-almond mixture evenly into apple cavities.

4 In bowl combine apricot nectar, vanilla and nutmeg. Pour around apples. Tightly cover with foil. Bake in preheated oven for 40 minutes. Remove foil. Bake for 25 to 30 minutes longer or until apples are tender, occasionally spooning liquid over apples. Cool slightly.

5 Transfer apples to serving dishes. Serve warm or chilled. Top with yogurt (if desired).

NUTRITION FACTS PER SERVING Calories: 230; **Calories from Fat:** 35; **Total Fat:** 4g; **Saturated Fat:** 0g; **Trans Fat:** 0g; **Cholesterol:** 0mg; **Sodium:** 5mg; **Total Carbohydrate:** 52g; **Dietary Fiber:** 7g; **Sugars:** 32g; **Protein:** 3g

Gingered Pear AND Cranberry Crumble

SERVES 9

4 medium pears, cored and thinly sliced (about 9 cups)

½ cup dried cranberries

½ cup firmly packed brown sugar

⅓ cup whole-wheat flour

3 tablespoons finely chopped crystallized ginger

½ teaspoon cinnamon

½ teaspoon vanilla

1 cup **Kellogg's® Special K®** Vanilla Almond cereal

2 tablespoons butter or margarine, melted

3 cups frozen low-fat vanilla yogurt (optional)

This fruit crisp combines fresh fall pears and dried cranberries, flavors them with spicy-sweet candied ginger, then covers them with a topping based on **Special K** cereal.

1 Preheat oven to 375°F.

2 In 8 x 8 x 2-inch baking dish toss together pears, cranberries, 2 tablespoons of the brown sugar, 2 tablespoons of the whole-wheat flour, ginger, cinnamon and vanilla.

3 In small bowl combine remaining brown sugar, remaining whole-wheat flour and **Special K** Vanilla Almond cereal. Drizzle with butter. Mix until combined. Sprinkle over fruit mixture. Bake in preheated oven for 25 minutes or until fruit is tender.

4 Serve warm with scoops of frozen yogurt, if desired.

Make it your own

Baked desserts featuring fruit with a crunchy crumb topping, crumbles can be among the most satisfying, healthy desserts—and they're easy to make.

Apple Crisp Replace the pears with apples such as Granny Smiths

Apple-Pear Crisp Use a mixture of apples and pears

Dried fruit variations In place of the dried cranberries, try seedless brown or golden raisins, diced dried apricots, or a mixture of your favorite dried fruits

NUTRITION FACTS PER SERVING Calories: 170; Calories from Fat: 25; Total Fat: 3g; Saturated Fat: 2g; Trans Fat: 0g; Cholesterol: 6mg; Sodium: 30mg; Total Carbohydrate: 37g; Dietary Fiber: 4g; Sugars: 25g; Protein: 1g

Individual Mango Buckles

SERVES 8

1¼ cups plus 1 tablespoon all-purpose flour

½ cup sugar

½ teaspoon baking powder

½ teaspoon baking soda

¼ teaspoon salt

¼ teaspoon nutmeg

⅔ cup nonfat plain yogurt

¼ cup refrigerated fat-free egg product

2 tablespoons vegetable oil

½ teaspoon vanilla

1 medium mango, peeled, seeded and finely chopped (about 1 cup)

2 tablespoons flaked coconut

2 cups frozen low-fat or nonfat vanilla yogurt (optional)

A low-fat, modern take on an old-fashioned baked dessert, these individual cakes studded with bits of fresh mango will win rave reviews from family and friends alike.

1 Preheat oven to 350°F.

2 Meanwhile, in large bowl stir together 1¼ cups flour, sugar, baking powder, baking soda, salt and nutmeg. Set aside.

3 In small bowl combine yogurt, egg product, oil and vanilla. Add to flour mixture. Stir just until moistened.

4 Toss mango with 1 tablespoon flour. Fold into batter. Portion evenly into eight ¾-cup ramekins or custard cups coated with cooking spray. Sprinkle with coconut. Place on baking sheet. Bake in preheated oven for 23 to 27 minutes or until toothpick inserted near center comes out clean. Serve warm with frozen yogurt, if desired.

Make it your own

Traditional desserts named for their appealing, uneven, golden-brown surfaces, buckles are made by folding fresh fruit into a cake batter and topping it with a sprinkling of crumbs, nuts or coconut flakes. Try these variations:

- Substitute other tropical fruit for the mango such as fresh pineapple or papaya

- Replace the mango with summer fruit, such as blueberries or pitted cherries

- In place of the coconut, substitute the crumble topping on page 215 or sliced almonds

NUTRITION FACTS PER SERVING Calories: 180; **Calories from Fat:** 35; **Total Fat:** 4g; **Saturated Fat:** 0.5g; **Trans Fat:** 0g; **Cholesterol:** 0mg; **Sodium:** 220mg; **Total Carbohydrate:** 33g; **Dietary Fiber:** 1g; **Sugars:** 18g; **Protein:** 4g

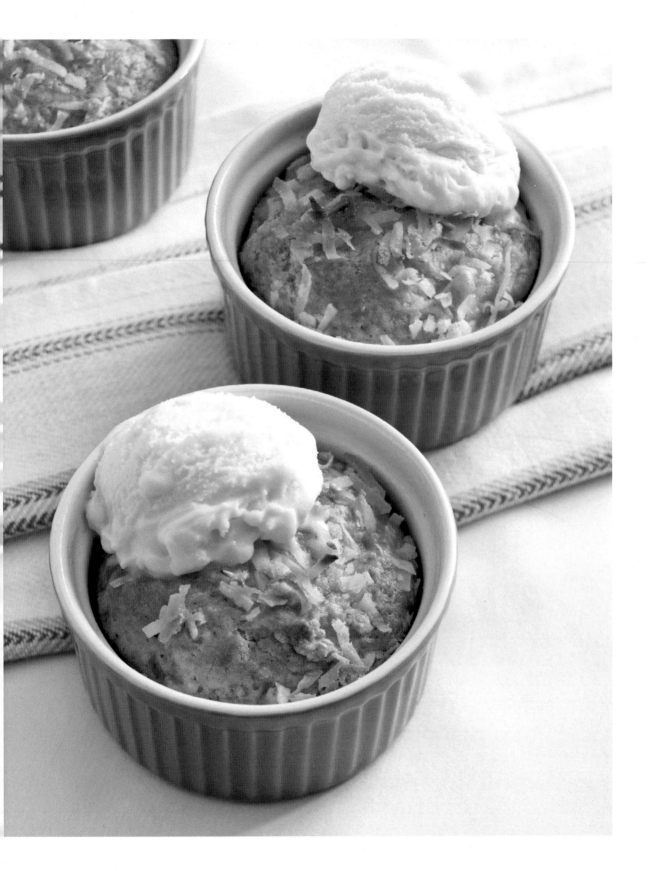

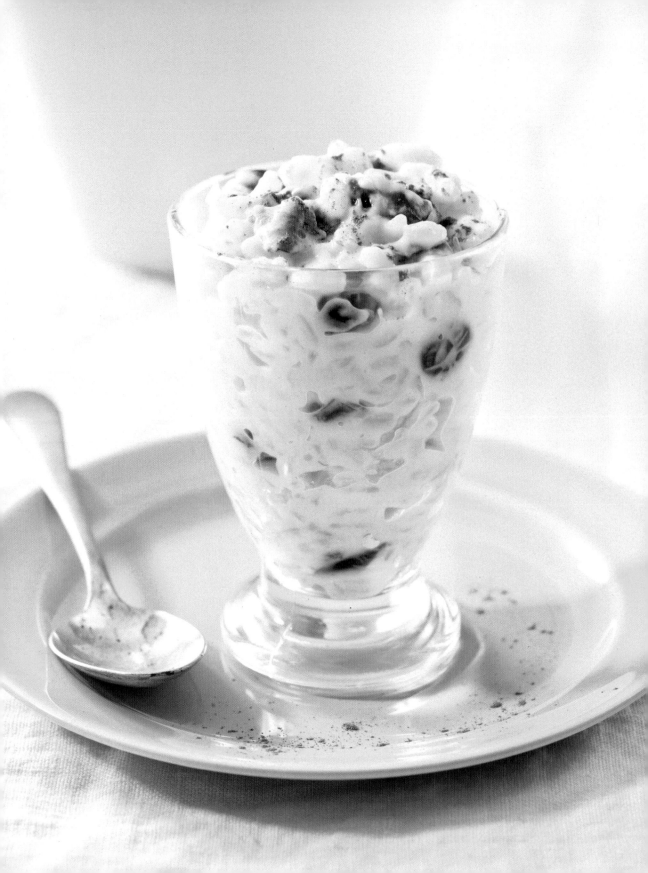

Rice Pudding WITH Dried Fruit

SERVES 6

1½ cups water

⅛ teaspoon salt

¾ cup uncooked Arborio rice

½ cup sugar

4 teaspoons cornstarch

2 cups reduced-fat (2%) milk

½ cup mixed dried fruit pieces

2 egg yolks

2 teaspoons butter or margarine

1 teaspoon vanilla

Ground cinnamon

This version of a dessert classic uses reduced-fat milk instead of the typical cream. The dried fruit adds flavor, color and texture for a satisfying finish to any meal.

1 In heavy medium saucepan combine water and salt. Bring to boiling. Stir in rice. Reduce heat. Simmer, covered, for 18 to 23 minutes or until water is absorbed.

2 Meanwhile, in medium bowl stir together sugar and cornstarch. Stir in milk and dried fruit. Stir milk mixture into hot rice. Bring mixture to boiling, stirring constantly.

3 Put egg yolks in mixing bowl and beat slightly. Stir about 1 cup of the hot rice mixture into yolks. Return all to saucepan and stir well. Cook over medium heat until just beginning to boil, stirring constantly. Remove from heat. Stir in butter and vanilla.

4 Spoon pudding into dessert dishes. Sprinkle with cinnamon. Serve pudding warm or chilled.

Make it your own

Although egg yolks, used to help thicken and enrich this low-fat dessert, are high in cholesterol, they generally don't impact blood cholesterol levels as much as do eating saturated fats and not exercising regularly. Egg yolks also provide far more iron, phosphorous, B vitamins and other nutrients than are found in egg whites alone.

NUTRITION FACTS PER SERVING Calories: 270; **Calories from Fat:** 40; **Total Fat:** 4.5g; **Saturated Fat:** 0g; **Trans Fat:** 0g; **Cholesterol:** 80mg; **Sodium:** 120mg; **Total Carbohydrate:** 51g; **Dietary Fiber:** 2g; **Sugars:** 28g; **Protein:** 6g

Streusel Dessert Squares

SERVES 16

3 cups **Kellogg's®
Special K®** Red
Berries cereal

1½ cups all-purpose flour

¾ cup firmly packed
brown sugar

¼ teaspoon salt

1 teaspoon ground
cinnamon

¼ cup butter or
margarine, cold

3 tablespoons
cold water

Butter-flavored
cooking spray

1 can (12 ounces)
strawberry or
raspberry pie filling

These deceptively low-fat treats feature a crust made from **Special K** Red Berries cereal and berry pie filling topping. Thanks to the prepared ingredients, they're easy to make.

1 Preheat oven to 325°F.

2 In large mixing bowl, combine **Special K** Red Berries cereal, flour, sugar, salt and cinnamon. Using pastry blender, cut in butter until cereal is crushed and mixture is like coarse crumbs. Stir in water. Remove 1½ cups crumb mixture, reserving for topping. Press remaining crumb mixture evenly and firmly into bottom of 9 x 9 x 2-inch baking pan coated with cooking spray.

3 Bake in preheated oven about 15 minutes or until lightly browned. Spread pie filling over hot crust and sprinkle evenly with reserved crumbs. Return to oven and bake 35 minutes longer or until top is golden brown. Cool completely in pan on wire rack. Cut into 16 squares, transfer to platter and serve.

NUTRITION FACTS PER SERVING Calories: 160; **Calories from Fat:** 25; **Total Fat:** 3g; **Saturated Fat:** 2g; **Trans Fat:** 0g; **Cholesterol:** 5mg; **Sodium:** 85mg; **Total Carbohydrate:** 32g; **Dietary Fiber:** 1g; **Sugars:** 18g; **Protein:** 2g

Caramel Apple Crisp

1 can (21 ounces)
apple pie filling

¼ cup dried cranberries

½ teaspoon apple
pie spice

Butter-flavored
cooking spray

⅓ cup fat-free
caramel topping

½ teaspoon butter
flavoring

3 cups **Kellogg's®
Special K®** cereal

Here, the comforting flavors of a favorite, old-fashioned treat are translated into an incredibly easy-to-make dessert using staples found in any supermarket.

1 Preheat oven to 350°F.

2 Combine apple pie filing, cranberries and apple pie spice. Place in shallow 2-quart baking dish coated with cooking spray. Set aside.

3 In medium size bowl, mix together caramel topping and butter flavoring. Toss with **Special K** cereal until thoroughly coated. Spread cereal mixture evenly over pie filling mixture.

4 Bake in preheated oven about 25 minutes or until cereal topping is golden brown. Serve warm.

Make it your own

Like its name suggests, a crisp is a fruit mixture baked with a crunchy topping. Using prepared fruit filling and **Special K** cereal topping, you can quickly and easily make your own variations. Try these to start:

- In place of the apple pie filling, try other canned fillings such as cherry, blueberry or peach. Or, use seedless raisins, dried cherries or chopped shelled nuts instead of the cranberries

- For variety in the topping, substitute other types of **Special K** cereal such as Cinnamon Pecan, Vanilla Almond, Blueberry or Red Berries

NUTRITION FACTS PER SERVING Calories: 230; **Calories from Fat:** 1; **Total Fat:** 0g; **Saturated Fat:** 0g; **Trans Fat:** 0g; **Cholesterol:** 0mg; **Sodium:** 200mg; **Total Carbohydrate:** 56g; **Dietary Fiber:** 2g; **Sugars:** 15g; **Protein:** 3g

Red Velvet Cupcakes

1⅓ cups all-purpose flour

1 tablespoon unsweetened cocoa powder

¼ teaspoon salt

¼ cup butter or margarine, softened

1 cup sugar

1 teaspoon vanilla

⅓ cup refrigerated fat-free egg product

5 teaspoons vegetable oil

2 teaspoons red food coloring

¾ cup low-fat buttermilk

1 teaspoon cider or white vinegar

¾ teaspoon baking soda

Powdered sugar

Tangy low-fat buttermilk and fat-free egg product make these deep-red, chocolaty, individual-serving cupcakes a guilt-free treat that everyone can enjoy.

1 Preheat oven to 350°F.

2 Meanwhile, in medium mixing bowl stir together flour, cocoa powder and salt. Set aside.

3 In large mixing bowl beat butter on medium speed of electric mixer until fluffy. Add sugar and vanilla. Beat until combined. Add egg product, half at a time, beating well after each addition. Add oil and food coloring. Beat on low speed until combined.

4 Alternately add flour mixture and buttermilk to beaten mixture, beating on low speed after each addition until just combined.

5 In small bowl stir together vinegar and baking soda. Add to batter. Beat until just combined. Portion evenly into twelve 2½-inch muffin-pan cups lined with foil baking cups.

6 Bake in preheated oven for 15 to 17 minutes or until toothpick inserted near center of a cupcake comes out clean. Cool in pan on wire rack for 5 minutes. Remove from pan. Cool completely. Sprinkle tops with powdered sugar and serve.

NUTRITION FACTS PER SERVING Calories: 180; Calories from Fat: 53; Total Fat: 6g; Saturated Fat: 3g; Trans Fat: 0g; Cholesterol: 8mg; Sodium: 188mg; Total Carbohydrate: 30g; Dietary Fiber: 0g; Sugars: 18g; Protein: 3g

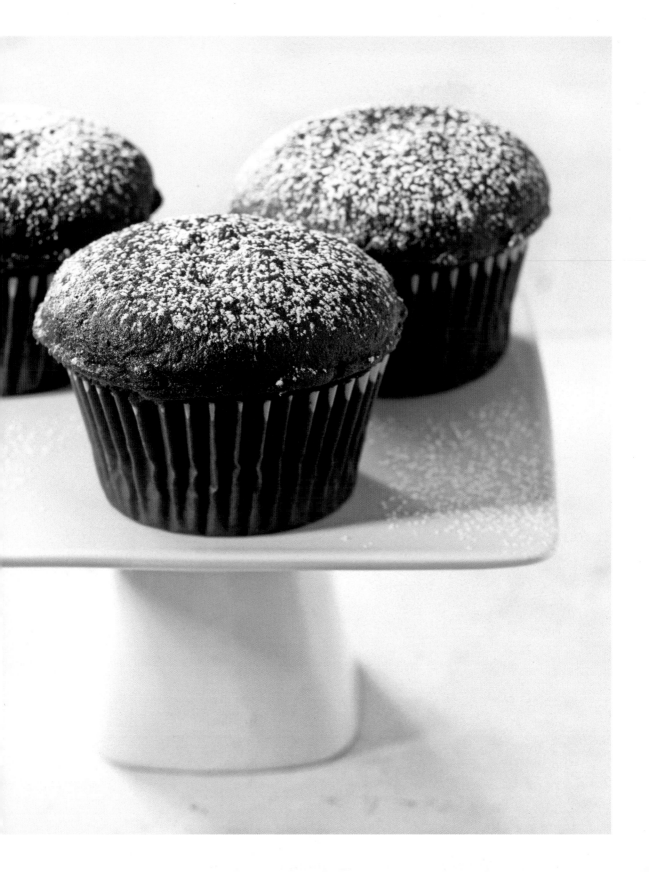

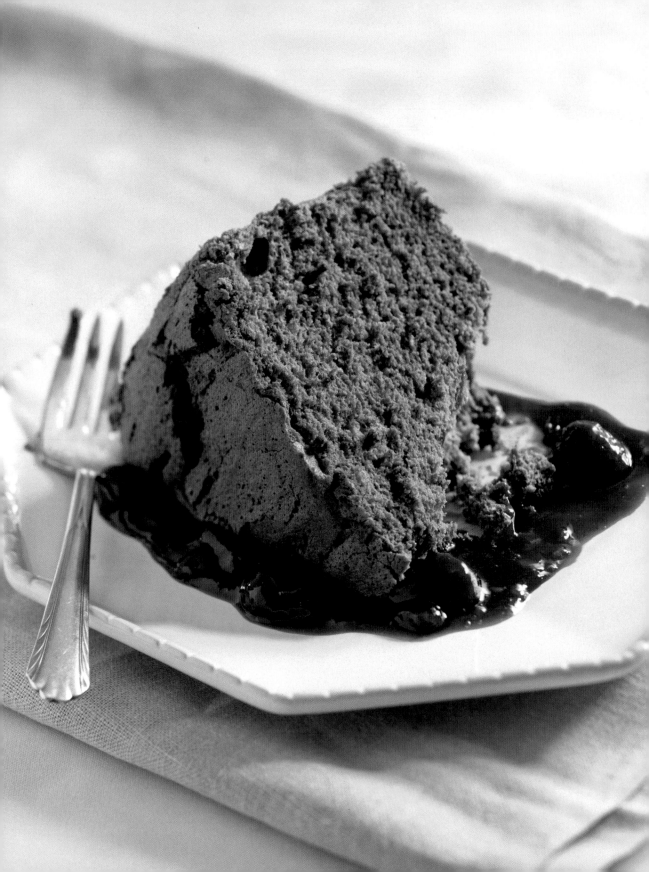

Dark Chocolate Angel Food Cake with Raspberry Sauce

SERVES 12

1½ cups sifted powdered sugar

1 cup sifted cake flour

½ cup unsweetened cocoa powder

12 egg whites

1½ teaspoons cream of tartar

1 teaspoon vanilla

1½ cups granulated sugar

2 packages (12 ounces each) frozen lightly sweetened raspberries, thawed

1 tablespoon cornstarch

Traditionally prepared with egg whites, angel food cake is a wonderful, low-fat dessert. A sauce made from pureed frozen raspberries is the perfect complement.

1 Preheat oven to 350°F and set oven rack on the lowest level.

2 Sift together powdered sugar, cake flour and cocoa powder. Repeat sifting. Set aside. In large mixer bowl beat egg whites, cream of tartar and vanilla on medium speed of electric mixer until soft peaks form. Gradually add 1 cup granulated sugar, beating until stiff peaks form.

3 Sift flour mixture, about one-fourth at a time, over egg white mixture. Fold by hand until combined. Repeat until all of the flour mixture is folded into egg white mixture.

4 Spread into ungreased 10-inch tube pan. Bake in preheated oven on lowest rack about 40 minutes or until cake springs back when lightly touched. Invert cake in pan on rack. Cool completely. Loosen cake from pan. Remove from pan.

5 Meanwhile, place 3 cups of the raspberries in food processor bowl. Cover and process until berries are nearly smooth. Strain puree through fine-mesh sieve. Discard seeds. (You should have about 1¼ cups raspberry puree.)

6 In small saucepan stir together ½ cup granulated sugar and cornstarch. Stir in raspberry puree. Cook and stir over medium heat until mixture boils and thickens slightly. Stir in remaining whole raspberries. Cover and refrigerate at least 1 hour before serving.

7 To serve, cut cake into wedges and transfer to individual serving plates. Spoon raspberry mixture alongside.

NUTRITION FACTS PER SERVING Calories: 260; Calories from Fat: 5; Total Fat: 0.5g; Saturated Fat: 0g; Trans Fat: 0g; Cholesterol: 0mg; Sodium: 55mg; Total Carbohydrate: 61g; Dietary Fiber: 2g; Sugars: 45g; Protein: 6g

Easy Key Lime Mousse
with Angel Food Cake

2 containers (6 ounces each) low-fat key lime yogurt

1 cup frozen reduced-fat nondairy whipped topping, thawed

4 cups angel food cake cubes (about ¼ of a 16-ounce cake)

1 tablespoon frozen limeade concentrate, thawed

4 fresh strawberries

You can prepare this refreshing, creamy lime dessert in a flash to make the end of any meal feel like a special occasion. Or enjoy it with a glass of iced tea for an afternoon snack.

1 In medium bowl fold together yogurt and whipped topping.

2 Arrange cake cubes in even layer in 4 dessert dishes. Drizzle limeade concentrate over top. Top with yogurt mixture. Garnish each serving with a strawberry.

Make it your own

The French word "mousse" means foam, which is a perfect description of this frothy-light dessert. Using different flavors of yogurt and angel food cake in the recipe can give you all kinds of tasty variations. Try these to get started:

- Other yogurt flavors that work well in this recipe include lemon, orange, strawberry and chocolate

- Look for prepared flavored angel food cake in your market. Or, try the dark chocolate recipe on page 225. You can also make angel food cake from a store-bought mix and flavor the batter with 1 teaspoon of your favorite flavor extract such as coffee or almond, or with 1 teaspoon of ground cinnamon or pumpkin pie spice

NUTRITION FACTS PER SERVING Calories: 210; Calories from Fat: 25; **Total Fat:** 3g; **Saturated Fat:** 2.5g; **Trans Fat:** 0g; **Cholesterol:** 5mg; **Sodium:** 180mg; **Total Carbohydrate:** 43g; **Dietary Fiber:** 0g; **Sugars:** 27g; **Protein:** 4g

Cream Cheese Pie
WITH Tropical Fruit Topping

SERVES 12

2 cups **Kellogg's®
Special K®** Red
Berries cereal
(crushed to 1 cup)

4 tablespoons seedless
strawberry jam

Butter-flavored
cooking spray

2 packages (8 ounces
each) nonfat cream
cheese, softened

¾ cup sliced ripe banana
(about 1 medium)

½ cup sugar

½ cup refrigerated
fat-free egg product

1 teaspoon vanilla

1 kiwi

2 cups chopped
fresh pineapple

Think of this as cheesecake without the guilt. **Special K** Red Berries cereal forms the crust, and nonfat cream cheese and ripe banana combine to make the creamy filling.

1 Preheat oven to 325°F.

2 In mixing bowl, combine **Special K** Red Berries cereal and 2 tablespoons of the jam. Spread on bottom and 1 inch up sides of 9-inch pie plate coated with cooking spray. Set aside.

3 In medium mixing bowl beat cream cheese, banana, sugar, egg product and vanilla on medium speed of electric mixer until smooth. Pour into prepared crust.

4 Bake in preheated oven about 40 minutes or until pie filling is set. Cool completely.

5 Peel kiwi, quarter lengthwise and slice. In small bowl combine kiwi, pineapple and remaining 2 tablespoons jam. Spread over cheese pie. Refrigerate, covered, until serving. Cut into wedges to serve.

NUTRITION FACTS PER SERVING Calories: 130; **Calories from Fat:** 0; **Total Fat:** 0g; **Saturated Fat:** 0g; **Trans Fat:** 0g; **Cholesterol:** 5mg; **Sodium:** 310mg; **Total Carbohydrate:** 27g; **Dietary Fiber:** 3g; **Sugars:** 19g; **Protein:** 7g

Fresh Blueberry-Ginger Fool

SERVES 4

¾ cup nonfat plain
Greek yogurt

2 tablespoons
powdered sugar

¼ teaspoon vanilla

1 cup frozen reduced-fat
nondairy whipped
topping, thawed

1½ cups fresh
blueberries

1½ teaspoons
granulated sugar

1 teaspoon grated
lemon zest

½ teaspoon grated
fresh ginger

Traditional English fool combines fruit puree and whipped cream. This low-fat version keeps the creamy texture and flavor with Greek yogurt and reduced-fat whipped topping.

1 In small bowl stir together yogurt, powdered sugar and vanilla. Fold in whipped topping.

2 Reserve about 12 blueberries for garnish. In shallow dish mash half of the remaining blueberries with potato masher. Stir in granulated sugar, ½ teaspoon of the lemon zest and ginger. Stir in remaining blueberries, leaving them whole.

3 Fold blueberry mixture into yogurt mixture. Spoon into dessert dishes. Garnish with reserved blueberries and remaining lemon zest.

Here's to your health

Though they may be small, blueberries are nutritional powerhouses. They are a source of antioxidants and fiber. Low in calories, very low in fat and packed with flavor, blueberries are among the smartest choices of fruit you can eat.

NUTRITION FACTS PER SERVING Calories: 120; Calories from Fat: 20; **Total Fat:** 2g; **Saturated Fat:** 2g; **Trans Fat:** 0g; **Cholesterol:** 0mg; **Sodium:** 15mg; **Total Carbohydrate:** 21g; **Dietary Fiber:** 1g; **Sugars:** 15g; **Protein:** 4g

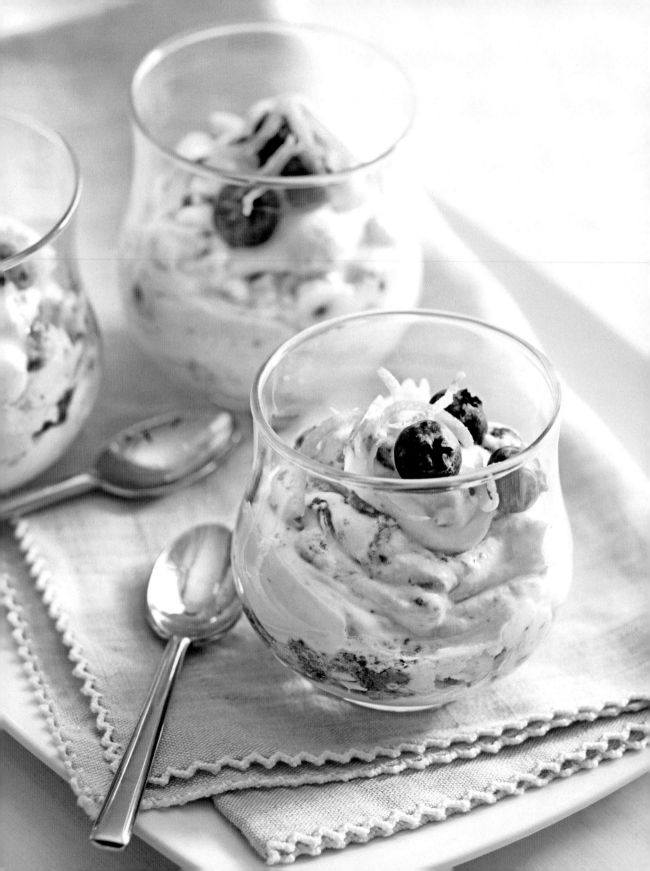

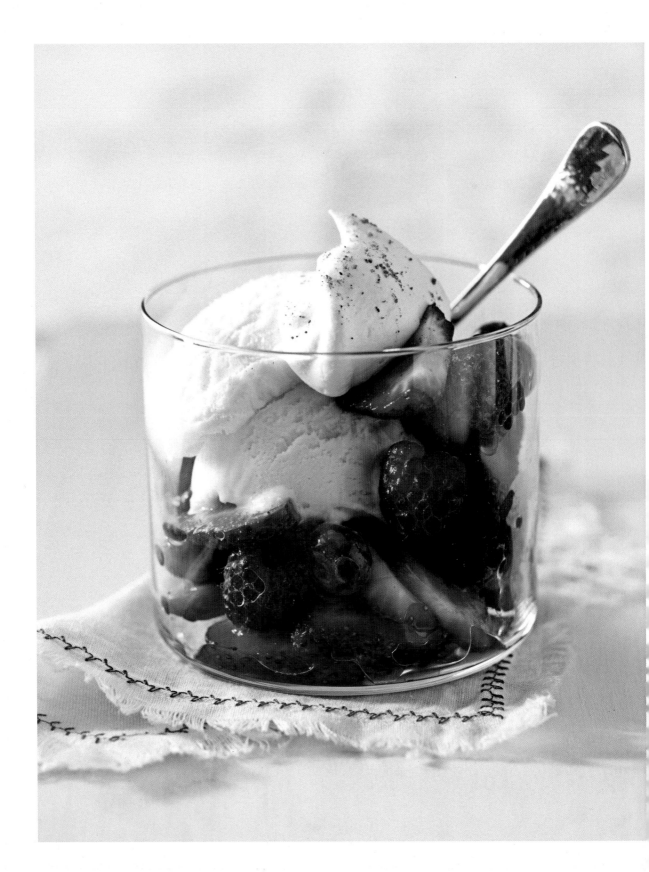

Frozen Yogurt
AND Berry Sundaes

SERVES 2

½ cup sliced fresh strawberries or red raspberries

½ cup fresh blueberries

1 tablespoon honey

1 teaspoon lemon juice

⅛ teaspoon nutmeg

⅔ cup low-fat or nonfat vanilla frozen yogurt

2 tablespoons frozen fat-free nondairy whipped topping, thawed

Just a hint of nutmeg complements the fresh blueberries and strawberries in this quick dessert. The recipe can be multiplied easily for larger gatherings.

1 In small bowl toss together strawberries, blueberries, honey, lemon juice and half of the nutmeg.

2 Scoop berry mixture into individual serving bowls. Top with frozen yogurt. Garnish each serving with dollop of whipped topping. Sprinkle each serving with remaining nutmeg.

Here's to your health

Lower in fat than traditional ice cream, frozen yogurt delivers a mixture of protein and carbohydrates, plus a generous amount of calcium in every serving. Look for products that contain the live cultures that transform milk into yogurt, which may provide health benefits.

NUTRITION FACTS PER SERVING Calories: 140; Calories from Fat: 20; **Total Fat:** 2.5g; **Saturated Fat:** 1g; **Trans Fat:** 0g; **Cholesterol:** 5mg; **Sodium:** 25mg; **Total Carbohydrate:** 30g; **Dietary Fiber:** 2g; **Sugars:** 23g; **Protein:** 2g

WEIGHT-MANAGEMENT JOURNAL

DATE _____   OVERALL CALORIE GOAL _____

What I ate today

MEAL 1
_____
_____ CALORIES _____

MEAL 2
_____
_____ CALORIES _____

MEAL 3
_____
_____ CALORIES _____

SNACK 4
_____
_____ CALORIES _____

My exercise today

ACTIVITY _____ TIME SPENT _____
ACTIVITY _____ TIME SPENT _____
ACTIVITY _____ TIME SPENT _____

My measurements today

WEIGHT _____ WAIST _____ HIPS _____ BUST _____ JEAN SIZE _____

How am I doing?

Write down here your thoughts on any triumphs, inspirations or even setbacks you may have had today that affected your personal weight-management journey, and what you learned from them.

_____
_____
_____

SEE PAGES 52-53 FOR A COMPLETE GUIDE TO USING THESE JOURNAL PAGES

WEIGHT-MANAGEMENT JOURNAL

DATE _____   OVERALL CALORIE GOAL _____

What I ate today

MEAL 1 _____
_____ CALORIES _____

MEAL 2 _____
_____ CALORIES _____

MEAL 3 _____
_____ CALORIES _____

SNACK 4 _____
_____ CALORIES _____

My exercise today

ACTIVITY _____   TIME SPENT _____

ACTIVITY _____   TIME SPENT _____

ACTIVITY _____   TIME SPENT _____

My measurements today

WEIGHT _____   WAIST _____   HIPS _____   BUST _____   JEAN SIZE _____

How am I doing?

Write down here your thoughts on any triumphs, inspirations or even setbacks you may have had today that affected your personal weight-management journey, and what you learned from them.

_____

_____

_____

SEE PAGES 52-53 FOR A COMPLETE GUIDE TO USING THESE JOURNAL PAGES

Index

weldonowen

415 Jackson Street, Suite 200, San Francisco, CA 94111
Telephone: 415 291 0100 Fax: 415 291 8841
www.wopublishing.com

Color separations by Embassy Graphics in Canada
Printed and bound in Canada by Transcontinental

First printed in 2011
10 9 8 7 6 5 4 3

Library of Congress Control Number: 2010941190

ISBN-13: 978-1-61628-062-8
ISBN-10: 1-61628-062-X

Weldon Owen wishes to thank the following people for their support in producing this book: **Managing Editor:** Norman Kolpas; **Recipes:** Marcia K. Stanley, MS, RD; **Text:** Serena Ball, MS, RD, Teaspoon Communications; **Copyediting:** Brenda Koplin; **Photographs:** Maren Caruso; **Food Styling:** Kim Kissling; **Illustrations:** Ann Field; **Index:** Elizabeth Parson

All recipes developed by Marcia K. Stanley except; pages 101, 134, 137, 140, 146, 161, 181, 184, 189 reprinted with permission from www.kelloggs.com

Every ingredient listed for use in recipe is included in the analysis. Optional ingredients, suggestions in recipe introductions or photographs are not included. Measurements are rounded for easier reading. Note: a serving for the recipe analysis is not necessarily a serving as defined by your daily food goals.

PHOTOGRAPHY CREDITS

All photographs by **Maren Caruso** except the following: **Bill Bettencourt** 25 (milk & dairy, meat & beans, oils); **Erika McConnell** 4 (top left, top right, bottom left); **Fotosearch:** UpperCut Images 4 (center); Ant Strack 4 (bottom right); **Getty:** Harrison Eastwood 2; Nancy R. Cohen 12; Fancy Photography 20; **Jupiter Images:** Jamie Grill 64; **Shutterstock:** AntiGerasim 27 (bread); Angelo Lorenzo 27 (pasta); Magone 27 (eggs); **Tucker + Hossler** 24 (vegetables); **Veer:** startoucher 25 (physical activity)

Additional photos courtesy of **specialk.com:** 16 (meal 1, meal 2, snack 4), 24 (grains), 25 (discretionary calories), 100, 135, 136, 141, 147, 160, 176, 180, 185, 188